THE SUPER EASY GALVESTON DIET COOKBOOK FOR BEGINNERS

1500 Days of Wholesome and Satisfying Recipes with a 28-Day Meal Plan for Menopausal Wellness to Boost Your Health | Full Color Edition

Marilyn R. Holland

Manufactured in the United States of America

Interior and Cover Designer: Danielle Rees

Art Producer: Brooke White

Editor: Aaliyah Lyons

Production Editor: Sienna Adams

Production Manager: Sarah Johnson

Photography: Michael Smith

TABLE OF CONTENTS

TABLE OF CONTENTS

TABLE OF CONTENTS

INTRODUCTION

I never envisioned myself narrating a menopause saga. Before this, life had sailed smoothly, but as my fifties dawned, menopause introduced itself with subtle yet persistent disturbances—a hot flash disrupting my workday, nights spent tossing instead of sleeping. These symptoms soon evolved from sporadic annoyances to constant, formidable presences in my daily life.

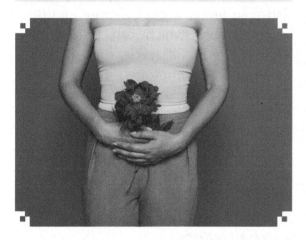

As I grappled with these changes, it wasn't just the physical symptoms that threw me; my once steady energy levels dipped, and my usual dietary habits no longer kept the scales at bay. I was battling a silent war against my body—a body that seemed foreign to me. The strategies I'd relied upon for years were now obsolete, leaving me both bewildered and determined to find a new path.

In my quest for answers, I discovered the Galveston diet. This wasn't merely another trend but a scientifically backed approach tailored for women like me, wrestling with the hormonal upheavals of menopause. Its foundation lies in combating inflammation and managing insulin resistance through a meticulously crafted regimen of whole foods, healthy fats, and optimal protein and carbohydrate balance.

with a blend of curiosity and hope, I embraced this new diet. My daily meals transformed into a palette of colorful vegetables, lean proteins like salmon and chicken, and heart-healthy fats from avocados and nuts. Intermittent fasting was introduced gradually, syncing perfectly with my lifestyle and reducing that overwhelming feeling of dietary restriction.

Months into this journey, the benefits were unmistakable. My weight was not only manageable but also decreasing steadily. My energy rebounded, sleep improved dramatically, and even my mood stabilized—allowing me to enjoy daily activities with a renewed spirit. The visible changes were complemented by the emotional uplift, painting my menopausal years in a more empowering light.

Motivated by my revitalization, I began to share this approach. The positive feedback from friends—who reported similar transformations—propelled me to reach a broader audience.

DEDICATION

Anne, where do I even begin? Thank you for being my rock and best friend for the past 30 years. Your support through every chapter of my life has been invaluable, and sharing your own experiences with me has always guided me through my toughest moments. Recently, recommending the Galveston diet was yet another instance of how you've positively impacted my life. Your thoughtful advice has set me on a path to better health and well-being. I'm deeply grateful for your friendship and everything you've done for me. Here's to many more years of sharing, caring, and unforgettable memories together!

CHAPTER 1: START THE GALVESTON DIET

UNDERSTANDING YOUR EVOLVING BODY

Navigating the intricate journey of menopause is akin to riding an emotional and physiological rollercoaster. This transformative phase can be daunting, but arming yourself with knowledge and effective management strategies can greatly alleviate discomfort and enhance your well-being. Let's delve deeper into the stages of menopause and explore targeted strategies to help you thrive during this pivotal time.

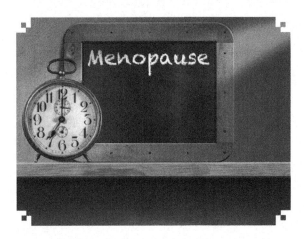

UNDERSTANDING THE STAGES OF MENOPAUSE

• PERIMENOPAUSE

Perimenopause serves as the introductory phase to menopause, marking the beginning of the body's gradual transition away from reproductive capability. This phase can start as early as your late 30s or as late as your 50s and is characterized by significant hormonal upheaval. Estrogen levels begin to surge and drop unpredictably, which can disrupt your regular menstrual cycle and introduce a variety of symptoms. These include intense hot flashes, disruptive night sweats, unpredictable mood swings, and sleep disturbances. Such symptoms are your body's way of signaling the winding down of your fertile years, setting the stage for menopause.

• MENOPAUSE

Menopause is officially diagnosed after you've gone a full year without a menstrual period. Entering this stage can bring a mix of relief and new health challenges. The most noticeable change is the cessation of menstrual cycles, but the decline in estrogen that defines menopause often leads to increased abdominal weight gain. This can be frustrating, as the weight is harder to shed due to a naturally slowing metabolism. Moreover, you may start to notice that your body reacts differently to the same foods you've always eaten, with changes in digestion and appetite frequently reported. This stage calls for a reassessment of dietary habits and physical activity routines to adapt to your body's new metabolic rate and nutritional needs.

• **POSTMENOPAUSE**

The postmenopausal phase encompasses the years following menopause, marking a new norm in your health landscape. While the tumultuous symptoms of earlier phases might lessen, this period brings its own set of health considerations. Decreased estrogen levels can lead to reduced bone density, making you more susceptible to osteoporosis. Similarly, changes in cholesterol levels and body composition can increase the risk of cardiovascular disease. It's crucial during this time to maintain regular health screenings and adopt lifestyle choices that support bone health, heart health, and overall vitality.

• **ANALYZING COMMON SYMPTOMS**

Throughout all these stages, some symptoms are more prevalent than others. Weight gain, especially around the midsection, and hot flashes are perhaps the most widely recognized menopausal symptoms. Hair may also

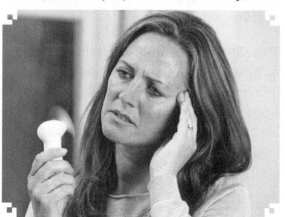

become thinner, drier, and less vibrant. Emotional fluctuations can resemble an unpredictable seesaw, making you feel as though you're losing control over your mood. Additionally, insomnia can transform what used to be a restful night's sleep into a fitful, intermittent experience. Recognizing these symptoms and understanding that they are normal can help you manage them more effectively.

MASTERING YOUR HORMONES

Understanding the intricate role of hormones in weight management is essential, particularly as your body undergoes the profound changes associated with menopause. It's a period marked not just by hormonal shifts but also by how these changes impact your overall health and weight. Let's debunk some prevalent myths about dieting, examine the hormonal influences on weight, and explore how targeted dietary strategies like the Galveston Diet can help address these imbalances effectively.

• **MYTHS AND REALITIES OF WEIGHT GAIN**

One common misconception is that weight gain during menopause is solely due to poor discipline or insufficient exercise. In truth, hormonal fluctuations play a critical role. As estrogen levels drop during menopause, women often see an increase in body fat, particularly around the abdomen. This change is not merely a superficial weight gain but a complex hormonal interaction that increases the risk of developing more serious health issues, such as heart disease and diabetes. Understanding that these changes are rooted in biology—not just calorie intake or exercise habits—is crucial for managing your health during menopause.

- **DETAILED HORMONAL ANALYSIS**

ESTROGEN

Estrogen is a key player in the female reproductive system but its influence extends far beyond. During menopause, as estrogen levels decline, there's a noticeable increase in abdominal fat. This type of fat is particularly concerning because it's associated with higher risks of heart disease and type 2 diabetes. Moreover, estrogen helps regulate how the body metabolizes starches and glucose. with lower estrogen levels, this metabolism can slow down, often leading to weight gain despite no significant change in diet.

INSULIN

Insulin is essential for regulating blood sugar levels by facilitating the uptake of glucose into cells for energy. However, as menopause progresses, the body's sensitivity to insulin can decrease, a condition known as insulin resistance. This resistance can cause higher levels of both glucose and insulin in the blood, contributing to weight gain and increasing the risk of diabetes. Managing insulin levels through diet and exercise is crucial during this time.

OTHER HORMONES: LEPTIN, GHRELIN, AND CORTISOL

Leptin and ghrelin are directly involved in appetite control. Leptin decreases appetite, while ghrelin increases it. Menopause can disrupt the balance between these hormones, often leading to increased hunger and a persistent feeling of not being full. Additionally, cortisol, the stress hormone, tends to rise during menopause. Elevated cortisol levels can lead to cravings for high-calorie foods, compounding weight gain issues. Balancing these hormones is key to maintaining a healthy weight during menopause.

EMBRACE TRANSFORMATION

- **INTERMITTENT FASTING**

Intermittent fasting (IF) is a dietary approach that cycles between periods of eating and fasting, focusing more on when you eat rather than what you eat. This method has gained popularity due to its simplicity and the significant health benefits it offers.

Rationale and Benefits of Intermittent Fasting

The rationale behind intermittent fasting is based on the theory that periods of fasting enable the body to rest and recover from constant digestion and nutrient assimilation. By doing this, IF taps into our body's innate mechanisms for optimizing energy metabolism.

One of the primary benefits of intermittent fasting is improved metabolic health. When you fast, the body lowers insulin levels, which facilitates fat burning. The drop in insulin that comes with fasting also increases insulin sensitivity, reducing the risk of type 2 diabetes. Moreover, fasting triggers a cellular response known as autophagy, where cells initiate a cleaning process, removing damaged cells and regenerating newer, healthier ones. This process is critical for cellular health and longevity.

Weight loss is another significant benefit of intermittent fasting. By limiting the window of time during which food is consumed, many find it easier to reduce calorie intake overall. Additionally, the hormonal changes from fasting help facilitate weight loss and fat loss rather than muscle loss.

- **IMPLEMENTING INTERMITTENT FASTING**

To implement intermittent fasting, start by choosing a fasting method that fits your lifestyle. Common approaches include:

- 16/8 Method: This involves fasting for 16 hours a day and eating all meals within an 8-hour window. For example, you might choose to eat between 12:00 pm and 8:00 pm.

- 5:2 Diet: In this method, you eat normally five days a week and reduce your calorie intake to about 500-600 calories on the other two days.

- Eat-Stop-Eat: This involves a 24-hour fast once or twice a week.

Beginners should start with a less restrictive regimen, such as the 16/8 method, and gradually extend the fasting period as they become more comfortable. It's important to consume balanced, nutritious meals during eating periods and stay hydrated with water, herbal teas, or black coffee during fasting periods.

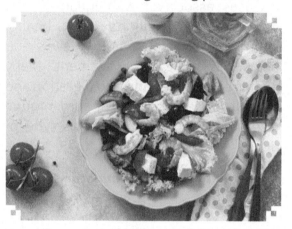

- **ANTI-INFLAMMATORY NUTRITION**

Anti-inflammatory nutrition focuses on consuming foods that help reduce chronic inflammation in the body, a root cause of numerous diseases including heart disease, diabetes, and arthritis. This approach to eating not only helps manage existing inflammatory conditions but also boosts overall health and prevents various health issues.

Rationale and Benefits of Anti-Inflammatory Nutrition

Chronic inflammation is an underlying factor in many serious health conditions. It can be triggered by various factors, including stress, lack of exercise, and particularly, a diet high in processed foods, sugars, and saturated fats. An anti-inflammatory diet counters this by including foods rich in antioxidants, fiber, and healthy fats, which help reduce inflammatory responses.

The benefits of adopting an anti-inflammatory diet are substantial. Primarily, it helps reduce the risk of chronic diseases associated with inflammation. Additionally, it supports heart health, improves mood, boosts energy levels, and helps with weight management. Many people also notice improved digestion and a reduction in symptoms of autoimmune diseases when they follow this type of diet.

Implementing Anti-Inflammatory Nutrition

Implementing an anti-inflammatory diet involves several straightforward steps:

Incorporate Plenty of Fruits and Vegetables: Aim for a variety of colors in your diet, as these often indicate a high antioxidant content which is crucial for reducing inflammation. Berries, leafy greens, and other brightly colored fruits and vegetables are excellent choices.

- Choose Whole Grains over Refined: Whole grains like oatmeal, brown rice, and whole-wheat bread are high in fiber, which can help to lower inflammation levels.

- Include Healthy Fats: Foods high in omega-3 fatty acids, such as salmon, flaxseeds, and walnuts, are particularly good for fighting inflammation. Olive oil is also a key component of an anti-inflammatory diet.

- Spice It Up: Many herbs and spices, including turmeric and ginger, have strong anti-inflammatory properties.

- Avoid Pro-inflammatory Foods: Reduce intake of processed foods, red meats, and foods high in refined sugars and unhealthy fats.

- **FUEL REFOCUS**

Fuel Refocus is a dietary strategy that emphasizes shifting away from a high-carbohydrate diet to one richer in proteins and healthy fats. This shift is based on the understanding that not all calories are created equal—different types of foods have varying effects on hunger, hormones, and how calories are burned.

Rationale and Benefits of Fuel Refocus

The traditional Western diet tends to be high in carbohydrates, particularly refined carbs and sugars, which can lead to spikes in blood sugar and insulin levels. These spikes are not only associated with increased fat storage but also with swings in energy levels and mood, and long-term, they can lead to insulin resistance and diabetes.

Refocusing your fuel sources towards proteins and healthy fats helps stabilize blood sugar levels, reduce insulin spikes, and increase satiety after meals. Protein is essential for building and repairing tissues and can also aid in weight loss by increasing metabolic rate and reducing appetite. Healthy fats,

such as those found in avocados, nuts, seeds, and oily fish, provide sustained

energy and support cell function, brain health, and the absorption of fat-soluble vitamins.

- **IMPLEMENTING FUEL REFOCUS**

To implement a Fuel Refocus strategy in your diet, consider the following steps:

- **Increase Protein Intake:** Include a source of high-quality protein at every meal. This could be from animal sources like chicken, fish, or eggs, or plant-based sources such as lentils, beans, and tofu.

- **Incorporate Healthy Fats:** Add fats that provide omega-3 and omega-6 fatty acids to your diet. Options include nuts, seeds, avocados, and fatty fish like salmon. Cooking with oils like olive or coconut oil can also help.

- **Reduce Refined Carbs:** Cut down on foods high in refined sugars and starches. Replace them with whole grains, such as quinoa, whole oats, and brown rice, which have a lower impact on blood sugar.

- **Eat Whole Foods:** Focus on whole, unprocessed foods, which naturally contain a balanced mix of macros and are less likely to cause inflammation and spikes in blood sugar.

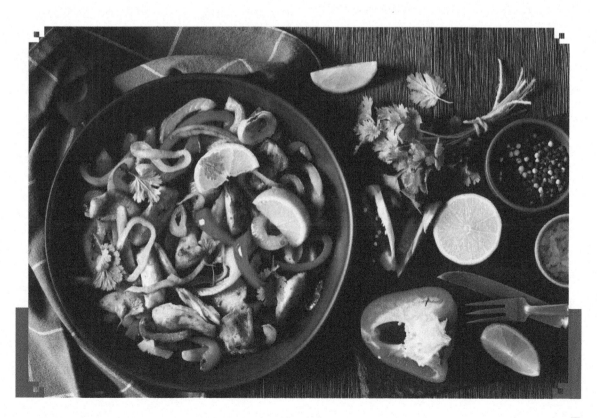

GALVESTON DIET SHOPPING LIST CHART

Category	Food Items
Proteins	Chicken breast, salmon, turkey, eggs, Greek yogurt, tofu, lean beef
Healthy Fats	Avocados, almonds, walnuts, flaxseeds, olive oil, coconut oil
Vegetables	Spinach, kale, broccoli, Brussels sprouts, bell peppers, sweet potatoes
Fruits	Berries (blueberries, strawberries), apples, oranges, kiwi
Whole Grains	Quinoa, brown rice, whole oats, whole-grain pasta
Dairy & Alternatives	Almond milk, cashew milk, feta cheese, cheddar cheese
Herbs & Spices	Turmeric, ginger, garlic, cinnamon, black pepper
Miscellaneous	Green tea, dark chocolate (70% or higher), nutritional yeast

TIPS FOR USING YOUR SHOPPING LIST:

- **Prioritize Fresh and Whole Foods:** Focus on buying fresh vegetables and fruits, and choose whole or minimally processed grains.

- **Consider Organic:** Where possible, opt for organic products to minimize exposure to pesticides and chemicals, which can contribute to inflammation.

- **Plan for Variety:** Make sure to include a variety of foods within each category to ensure a wide range of nutrients and to keep your meals interesting.

- **Check for Seasonality:** Purchase seasonal fruits and vegetables as they tend to be fresher and more affordable.

In conclusion, the Galveston Diet offers a transformative approach to health and wellness, focusing on anti-inflammatory foods, strategic eating patterns, and balanced nutrition to combat the challenges of menopause and aging. This cookbook is designed to guide you through making dietary choices that not only enhance your overall health but also empower you to lead a vibrant, energetic life. Whether you are new to this way of eating or looking to refine your dietary habits, the recipes and tips provided herein will support you on your journey to wellness, ensuring that each meal brings you one step closer to achieving your health goals.

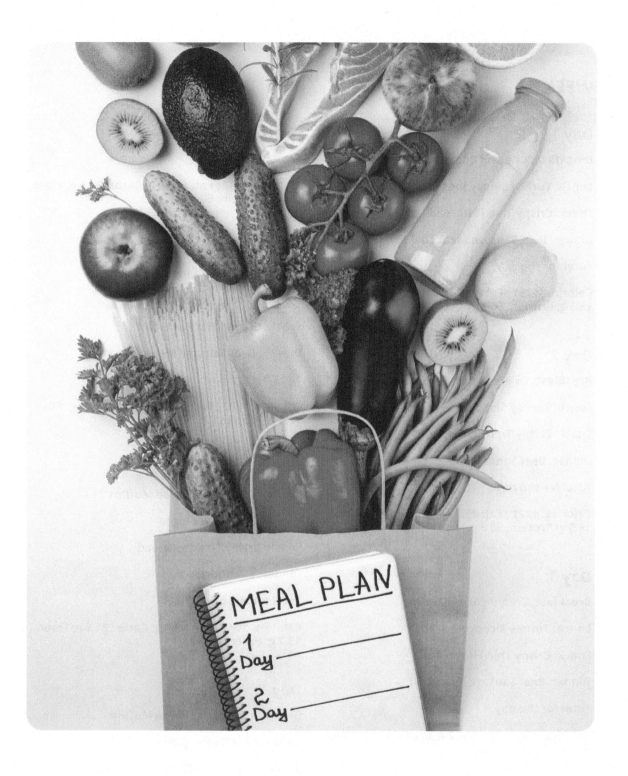

CHAPTER 2: 4-WEEK MEAL PLAN

WEEK 1

Day 1:

Breakfast: **Kale and Banana Smoothie**

Lunch: **Turkey Sloppy Joes**

Snack: **Crispy Thin Flatbread**

Dinner: **Beef Sausage Meat Loaf**

Total for the day:

Calories: **1221** ; Fat: **85.2 g**; Carbs: **64.4 g**; Fiber: **16.5 g**; Protein: **56.3 g**

Day 2:

Breakfast: **Kale and Banana Smoothie**

Lunch: **Turkey Sloppy Joes**

Snack: **Crispy Thin Flatbread**

Dinner: **Beef Sausage Meat Loaf**

Total for the day:

Calories: **1221** ; Fat: **85.2 g**; Carbs: **64.4 g**; Fiber: **16.5 g**; Protein: **56.3 g**

Day 3:

Breakfast: **Cream Cheese Muffins**

Lunch: **Turkey Sloppy Joes**

Snack: **Crispy Thin Flatbread**

Dinner: **Beef Sausage Meat Loaf**

Total for the day:

Calories: **1287** ; Fat: **104.2 g**; Carbs: **33.4 g**; Fiber: **12.5 g**; Protein: **60.3 g**

Day 4:

Breakfast: **Cream Cheese Muffins**

Lunch: **Turkey Sloppy Joes**

Snack: **Crispy Thin Flatbread**

Dinner: **Beef Sausage Meat Loaf**

Total for the day:

Calories: **1287** ; Fat: **104.2 g**; Carbs: **33.4 g**; Fiber: **12.5 g**; Protein: **60.3 g**

Day 5:

Breakfast: **Cream Cheese Muffins**

Lunch: **Turkey Sloppy Joes**

Snack: **Crispy Thin Flatbread**

Dinner: **Beef Sausage Meat Loaf**

Total for the day:

Calories: **1287** ; Fat: **104.2 g**; Carbs: **33.4 g**; Fiber: **12.5 g**; Protein: **60.3 g**

Day 6:

Breakfast: **Cream Cheese Muffins**

Lunch: **Cauliflower Rice**

Snack: **Crispy Thin Flatbread**

Dinner: **Cauliflower Rice**

Total for the day:

Calories: **1042** ; Fat: **92.6 g**; Carbs: **31.6 g**; Fiber: **15.7 g**; Protein: **26.5 g**

Day 7:

Breakfast: **Cream Cheese Muffins**

Lunch: **Cauliflower Rice**

Snack: **Crispy Thin Flatbread**

Dinner: **Cauliflower Rice**

Total for the day:

Calories: **1042** ; Fat: **92.6 g**; Carbs: **31.6 g**; Fiber: **15.7 g**; Protein: **26.5 g**

WEEK 2

Day 1:

Breakfast: Granola Cups with Yogurt

Lunch: Salt and Pepper Ribs

Snack: Jerk Chicken

Dinner: Salt and Pepper Ribs

Total for the day:

Calories: 1281; Fat: 85 g; Carbs: 16 g; Fiber: 3.5 g; Protein: 108.6 g

Day 2:

Breakfast: Granola Cups with Yogurt

Lunch: Salt and Pepper Ribs

Snack: Jerk Chicken

Dinner: Salt and Pepper Ribs

Total for the day:

Calories: 1281; Fat: 85 g; Carbs: 16 g; Fiber: 3.5 g; Protein: 108.6 g

Day 3:

Breakfast: Granola Cups with Yogurt

Lunch: Salt and Pepper Ribs

Snack: Jerk Chicken

Dinner: Salt and Pepper Ribs

Total for the day:

Calories: 1281; Fat: 85 g; Carbs: 16 g; Fiber: 3.5 g; Protein: 108.6 g

Day 4:

Breakfast: Granola Cups with Yogurt

Lunch: Salt and Pepper Ribs

Snack: Jerk Chicken

Dinner: Salt and Pepper Ribs

Total for the day:

Calories: 1281; Fat: 85 g; Carbs: 16 g; Fiber: 3.5 g; Protein: 108.6 g

Day 5:

Breakfast: Granola Cups with Yogurt

Lunch: Vegetarian Pad Thai

Snack: Jerk Chicken

Dinner: Vegetarian Pad Thai

Total for the day:

Calories: 823; Fat: 52 g; Carbs: 29 g; Fiber: 9.5 g; Protein: 52 g

Day 6:

Breakfast: Granola Cups with Yogurt

Lunch: Vegetarian Pad Thai

Snack: Jerk Chicken

Dinner: Vegetarian Pad Thai

Total for the day:

Calories: 823; Fat: 52 g; Carbs: 29 g; Fiber: 9.5 g; Protein: 52 g

Day 7:

Breakfast: Granola Cups with Yogurt

Lunch: Vegetarian Pad Thai

Snack: Jerk Chicken

Dinner: Vegetarian Pad Thai

Total for the day:

Calories: 823; Fat: 52 g; Carbs: 29 g; Fiber: 9.5 g; Protein: 52 g

WEEK 3

Day 1:

Breakfast: Spinach Frittata

Lunch: Hot and Spicy Tiger Prawns

Snack: Sweet Potato Chips

Dinner: Creamy Roasted Asparagus Salad

Total for the day:

Calories: 868; Fat: 52 g; Carbs: 51.4 g; Fiber: 9.6 g; Protein: 56.5 g

Day 2:

Breakfast: Spinach Frittata

Lunch: Hot and Spicy Tiger Prawns

Snack: Sweet Potato Chips

Dinner: Creamy Roasted Asparagus Salad

Total for the day:

Calories: 868; Fat: 52 g; Carbs: 51.4 g; Fiber: 9.6 g; Protein: 56.5 g

Day 3:

Breakfast: Spinach Frittata

Lunch: Hot and Spicy Tiger Prawns

Snack: Sweet Potato Chips

Dinner: Creamy Roasted Asparagus Salad

Total for the day:

Calories: 868; Fat: 52 g; Carbs: 51.4 g; Fiber: 9.6 g; Protein: 56.5 g

Day 4:

Breakfast: Spinach Frittata

Lunch: Hot and Spicy Tiger Prawns

Snack: Sweet Potato Chips

Dinner: Creamy Roasted Asparagus Salad

Total for the day:

Calories: 868; Fat: 52 g; Carbs: 51.4 g; Fiber: 9.6 g; Protein: 56.5 g

Day 5:

Breakfast: Sweet Potato Hash

Lunch: Hot and Spicy Tiger Prawns

Snack: Sweet Potato Chips

Dinner: Creamy Roasted Asparagus Salad

Total for the day:

Calories: 877; Fat: 42 g; Carbs: 84.4 g; Fiber: 14.6 g; Protein: 73.5 g

Day 6:

Breakfast: Sweet Potato Hash

Lunch: Hot and Spicy Tiger Prawns

Snack: Sweet Potato Chips

Dinner: Cilantro Garlic Pork Chops

Total for the day:

Calories: 947; Fat: 40.5 g; Carbs: 81.7 g; Fiber: 12.6 g; Protein: 96 g

Day 7:

Breakfast: Sweet Potato Hash

Lunch: Cilantro Garlic Pork Chops

Snack: Sweet Potato Chips

Dinner: Cilantro Garlic Pork Chops

Total for the day:

Calories: 977 ; Fat: 50 g; Carbs: 81 g; Fiber: 12 g; Protein: 82 g

WEEK 4

Day 1:

Breakfast: Egg Tart

Lunch: Creamy Chicken Pesto Pasta

Snack: Egg-Free Vanilla Spice Cookies

Dinner: Shrimp with Cinnamon Sauce

Total for the day:

Calories: 1220; Fat: 80 g; Carbs: 46.8 g; Fiber: 12.8 g; Protein: 85.3 g

Day 2:

Breakfast: Egg Tart

Lunch: Creamy Chicken Pesto Pasta

Snack: Egg-Free Vanilla Spice Cookies

Dinner: Shrimp with Cinnamon Sauce

Total for the day:

Calories: 1220; Fat: 80 g; Carbs: 46.8 g; Fiber: 12.8 g; Protein: 85.3 g

Day 3:

Breakfast: Egg Tart

Lunch: Creamy Chicken Pesto Pasta

Snack: Egg-Free Vanilla Spice Cookies

Dinner: Shrimp with Cinnamon Sauce

Total for the day:

Calories: 1220; Fat: 80 g; Carbs: 46.8 g; Fiber: 12.8 g; Protein: 85.3 g

Day 4:

Breakfast: Egg Tart

Lunch: Creamy Chicken Pesto Pasta

Snack: Egg-Free Vanilla Spice Cookies

Dinner: Shrimp with Cinnamon Sauce

Total for the day:

Calories: 1220; Fat: 80 g; Carbs: 46.8 g; Fiber: 12.8 g; Protein: 85.3 g

Day 5:

Breakfast: Egg Tart

Lunch: Creamy Chicken Pesto Pasta

Snack: Egg-Free Vanilla Spice Cookies

Dinner: Brussels Sprout Slaw

Total for the day:

Calories: 1139; Fat: 77 g; Carbs: 71.8 g; Fiber: 19.8 g; Protein: 52.3 g

Day 6:

Breakfast: Egg Tart

Lunch: Creamy Chicken Pesto Pasta

Snack: Egg-Free Vanilla Spice Cookies

Dinner: Brussels Sprout Slaw

Total for the day:

Calories: 1139; Fat: 77 g; Carbs: 71.8 g; Fiber: 19.8 g; Protein: 52.3 g

Day 7:

Breakfast: Egg Tart

Lunch: Brussels Sprout Slaw

Snack: Egg-Free Vanilla Spice Cookies

Dinner: Brussels Sprout Slaw

Total for the day:

Calories: 1042 ; Fat: 73 g; Carbs: 73.8 g; Fiber: 26.8 g; Protein: 38.3 g

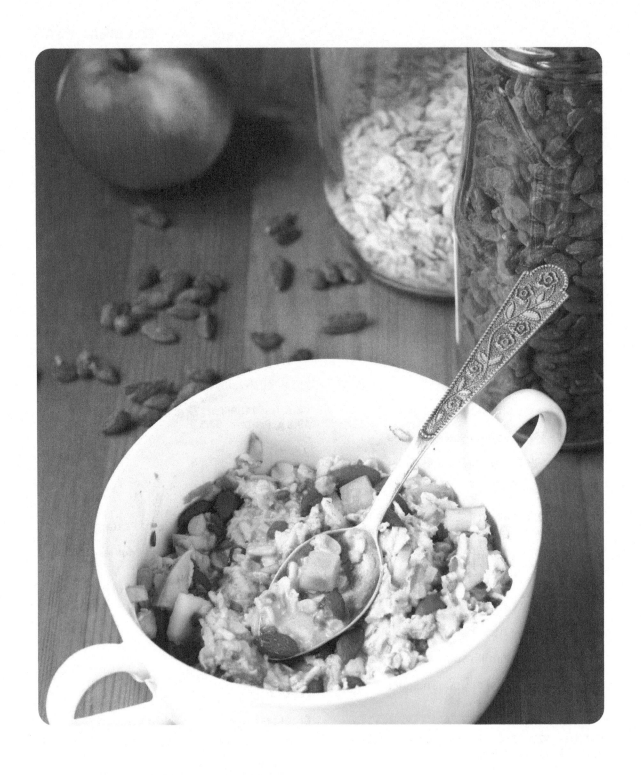

CHAPTER 3: BREAKFAST AND SMOOTHIES

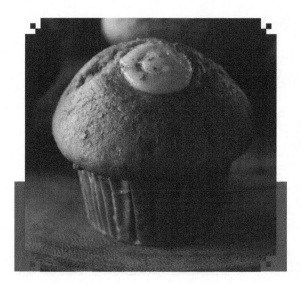

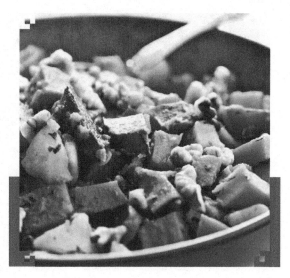

CREAM CHEESE MUFFINS

Prep time: **10 minutes** | Cook time: **10 minutes** | Serves **6**

- 4 tablespoons melted butter, plus more for the muffin tin
- 1 cup almond flour
- ¾ tablespoon baking powder
- 2 large eggs, lightly beaten
- 2 ounces cream cheese mixed with 2 tablespoons heavy (whipping) cream
- Handful shredded Mexican blend cheese

1. Preheat the oven to 400°F. Coat six cups of a muffin tin with butter.
2. In a small bowl, mix together the almond flour and baking powder.
3. In a medium bowl, mix together the eggs, cream cheese–heavy cream mixture, shredded cheese, and 4 tablespoons of the melted butter.
4. Pour the flour mixture into the egg mixture, and beat with a hand mixer until thoroughly mixed.
5. Pour the batter into the prepared muffin cups.
6. Bake for 12 minutes, or until golden brown on top, and serve.

Per Serving

Calories: **247** | Fat: **23g** | Carbs: **6g** | Fiber: **2g** | Protein: **8g**

SWEET POTATO HASH

Prep time: **15 minutes** | Cook time: **15 minutes** | Serves **4**

- 2 tablespoons coconut oil
- ½ onion, sliced thin
- 1 cup sliced mushrooms
- 1 garlic clove, sliced thin
- 2 large sweet potatoes, cooked and cut into ½-inch cubes
- 1 cup finely chopped Swiss chard
- ½ cup vegetable broth
- 1 teaspoon salt
- ¼ teaspoon freshly ground pepper
- 1 tablespoon chopped fresh thyme
- 1 tablespoon chopped fresh sage

1. In a large skillet over high heat, melt the coconut oil.
2. Add the onion, mushrooms, and garlic. Sauté for about 8 minutes, or until the onions and mushrooms are tender.
3. Add the sweet potatoes, Swiss chard, and vegetable broth. Cook for 5 minutes.
4. Stir in the salt, pepper, thyme, and sage.

Per Serving

Calories: **212** | Fat: **7g** | Carbs: **35g** | Fiber: **6g** | Protein: **30g**

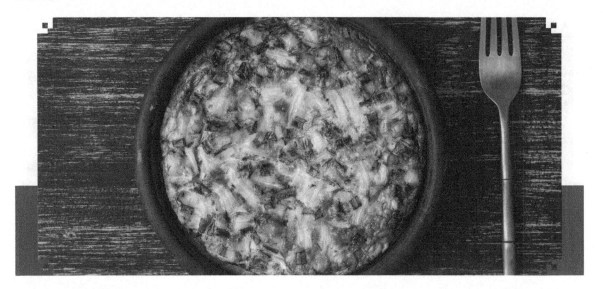

PEACHY MINT PUNCH

Prep time: **15 minutes** | Cook time: **15 minutes** | Serves **4**

- 1 (10-ounce) bag frozen no-added-sugar peach slices, thawed
- 3 tablespoons freshly squeezed lemon juice
- 3 tablespoons raw honey or maple syrup
- 1 tablespoon lemon zest
- 2 cups coconut water
- 2 cups sparkling water
- 4 fresh mint sprigs, divided
- Ice

1. In a food processor, combine the peaches, lemon juice, honey, and lemon zest. Process until smooth.
2. In a large pitcher, stir together the peach purée and coconut water. Chill the mixture in the refrigerator.
3. When ready to serve, fill four large (16-ounce) glasses with ice. Add 1 mint sprig to each glass. Add about ¾ cup peach mixture to each glass and top each with sparkling water.

Per Serving

Calories: **81** | Fat: **0g** | Carbs: **18g** | Fiber: **1g** | Protein: **0g**

SPINACH & LEEK FRITTATA

Prep time: **5 minutes** | Cook time: **20 minutes** | Serves **4**

- 2 leeks (white and pale green parts only), thoroughly washed and finely chopped
- 2 tablespoons avocado oil
- 8 eggs
- ¾ teaspoon salt
- ½ teaspoon garlic powder
- ½ teaspoon dried basil
- 1 cup packed fresh baby spinach leaves, thoroughly washed and dried
- 1 cup sliced cremini mushrooms
- Freshly ground black pepper

1. Preheat the oven to 400°F.
2. In a large ovenproof skillet over medium-high heat, sauté the leeks in the avocado oil for about 5 minutes until soft.
3. In a medium bowl, whisk the eggs, salt, garlic powder, and basil. Add to the skillet with the leeks. Cook for 5 minutes, stirring frequently.
4. Stir in the spinach and mushrooms. Season with pepper. Transfer the skillet to the oven. Bake for 10 minutes, or until the eggs are firmly set.

Per Serving

Calories: **276** | Fat: **17g** | Carbs: **15g** | Fiber: **3g;** | Protein: **19g**

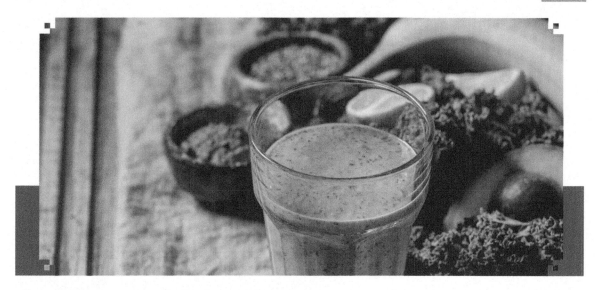

KALE AND BANANA SMOOTHIE

Prep time: **5 minutes** | Cook time: **15 minutes** | Serves **2**

- 2 cups unsweetened almond milk
- 2 cups kale, stemmed, leaves chopped
- 2 bananas, peeled

- 1 to 2 packets stevia, or to taste
- 1 teaspoon ground cinnamon
- 1 cup crushed ice

1. In a blender, combine the almond milk, kale, bananas, stevia, cinnamon, and ice. Blend until smooth.

Per Serving

Calories: **181** | Fat: **4g** | Carbs: **37g** | Fiber: **6g** | Protein: **4g**

EGG TART

Prep time: **20 minutes** | Cook time: **20 minutes** | Makes one 8-inch pie

- 1 cup Cheesy Yellow Sauce or Cauliflower Alfredo
- 1 baked Pie Crust
- 4 large eggs

- ¼ teaspoon fine Himalayan salt
- ¼ teaspoon ground black pepper
- 4 slices prosciutto di Parma

1. Spread the sauce evenly on the bottom of the baked pie crust. Crack the eggs over the sauce and sprinkle with the salt and pepper. Distribute the prosciutto slices around the eggs. Wrap the edges of the crust in aluminum foil so they do not burn.
2. Bake for 20 minutes, or until the egg whites are completely set. You can test this by gently shaking the pie to watch for a jiggle—when it doesn't move, it's done.
3. Remove from the oven and serve hot, or let cool and store in the refrigerator, covered, for up to 3 days. To reheat, cut into four large slices, cover each slice with foil, and bake in a preheated 300°F oven for 10 minutes.

Per Serving

Calories: **471** | Fat: **40.6g** | Carbs: **9.2g** | Fiber: **6.3g** | Protein: **19.1g**

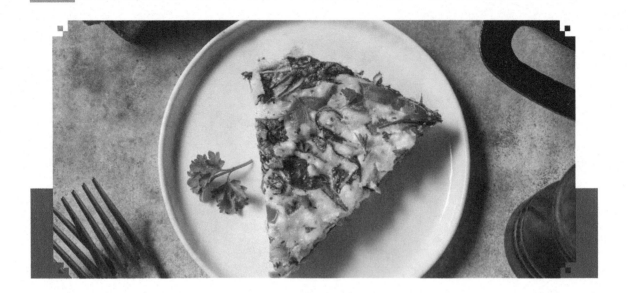

SPINACH FRITTATA

Prep time: 10 minutes | Cook time: 12 minutes | Serves 4

- 2 tablespoons extra-virgin olive oil
- 2 cups fresh baby spinach
- 8 eggs, beaten
- 1 teaspoon garlic powder
- ½ teaspoon sea salt
- ⅛ teaspoon freshly ground black pepper
- 2 tablespoons grated parmesan cheese

1. Preheat the broiler to high.
2. In a large ovenproof skillet (well-seasoned cast iron works well) over medium-high heat, heat the olive oil until it shimmers.
3. Add the spinach and cook for about 3 minutes, stirring occasionally.
4. In a medium bowl, whisk the eggs, garlic powder, salt, and pepper.Carefully pour the egg mixture over the spinach and cook the eggs for about 3 minutes until they begin to set around the edges.
5. Using a rubber spatula, gently pull the eggs away from the edges of the pan. Tilt the pan to let the uncooked egg flow into the edges. Cook for 2 to 3 minutes until the edges set.
6. Sprinkle with the parmesan cheese and put the skillet under the broiler. Broil for about 3 minutes until the top puffs.
7. Cut into wedges to serve.

Per Serving

Calories: 203 | Fat: 17g |Carbs: 2g | Fiber: <1g | Protein: 13g

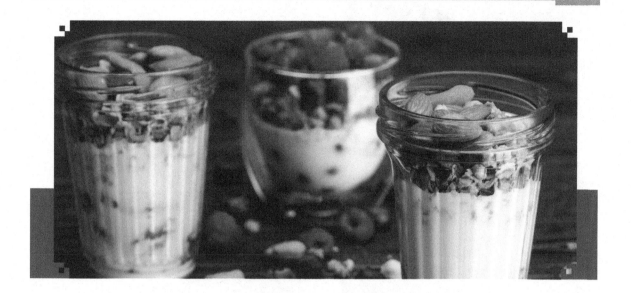

GRANOLA CUPS WITH YOGURT

Prep time: 10 minutes | Cook time: 10 minutes | Serves 12

- 1 cup rolled oats
- ½ cup almond flour
- 2 tablespoons coconut sugar
- ½ teaspoon baking soda
- ½ cup dried cranberries, blueberries, or goji berries
- ¼ cup pecans, chopped
- ¼ cup sliced almonds
- 2 tablespoons unsweetened dried coconut
- 4 tablespoons coconut oil, divided
- 3 tablespoons pure maple syrup
- 1 teaspoon vanilla extract
- 2 cups plain whole-milk yogurt

1. Preheat the oven to 325°F.
2. In a medium bowl, mix the oats, almond flour, coconut sugar, baking soda, dried berries, pecans, almonds, and coconut.
3. In a microwave-safe bowl, melt 3 tablespoons of coconut oil. Stir in the maple syrup and vanilla. Add the coconut oil-maple syrup to the oat mixture and stir well to combine.
4. Using the remaining 1 tablespoon of coconut oil, lightly coat the cups of a standard muffin tin.
5. Evenly divide the granola mixture among the cups, pressing it in to create a bowl shape in each cup. Bake for 10 minutes. Cool completely before carefully removing the cups.
6. Fill each cup with some of the yogurt and serve.

Per Serving

Calories: 183 | Fat: 12g | Carbs: 12g | Fiber: 3g; | Protein: 4g

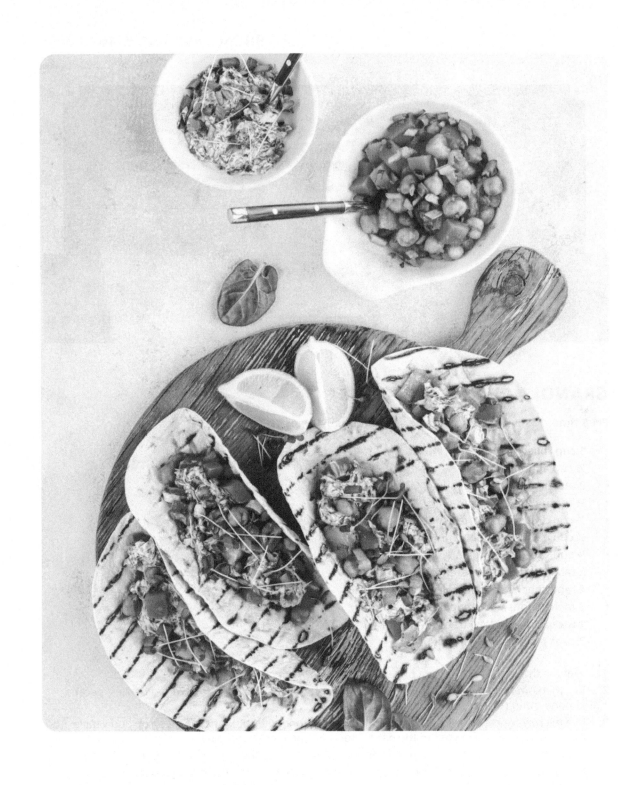

CHAPTER 4: SNACKS AND APPETIZERS

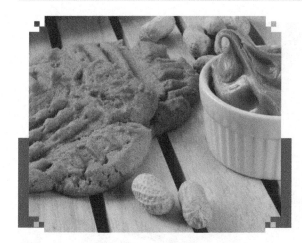

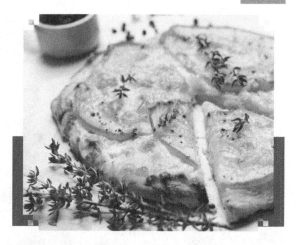

SALTED PEANUT BUTTER COOKIES

Prep time: **10 minutes** | **Cook time: 40 minutes** | **Serves 4**

- 1 cup all-natural peanut butter (no added sugar)
- 1 cup granulated erythritol–monk fruit blend; less sweet: ½ cup
- 8 tablespoons (1 stick) unsalted

- butter, at room temperature
- 1 large egg, at room temperature
- 1 cup finely milled almond flour
- 1 teaspoon baking powder
- ½ teaspoon sea salt

1. Preheat the oven to 350°F. Line the baking sheet with parchment paper.
2. In the large bowl, using an electric mixer on medium high, combine the peanut butter, erythritol–monk fruit blend, butter, and egg and mix until combined, stopping and scraping the bowl once or twice, as needed. Add the almond flour and baking powder. Mix on low until fully incorporated.
3. Using a small cookie scoop or spoon, place tablespoon-size cookies on the prepared baking sheet and flatten them with the tines of a fork to make a crisscross design. Sprinkle the tops with the salt. Bake for 10 to 12 minutes, until lightly browned around the edges.
4. Allow the cookies to cool completely before eating.
5. Carefully handle these cookies when storing because they can be very fragile. They will last in the refrigerator for up to 5 days or in the freezer for up to 3 weeks.

Per Serving

Calories: 360 | Fat: 32g | Carbs: 3g | Fiber: 2g | Protein: 11g

CRISPY THIN FLATBREAD

Prep time: 10 minutes | **Cook time: 20 minutes** | **Makes two 8-inch crusts**

- 4 large eggs, cold
- ½ cup coconut oil, melted
- ½ teaspoon fine Himalayan salt
- ⅓ cup coconut flour, plus more if needed

1. Preheat the oven to 400°F. Line a baking sheet with parchment paper.
2. In a small bowl, whisk the eggs as you slowly pour in the coconut oil—it will become creamy. Then add the salt and stir to combine. Add the coconut flour and fold until a loose dough forms
3. The density of coconut flour can vary from brand to brand. If the dough does not take shape, add more flour a teaspoon at a time, waiting at least 30 seconds before adding the next teaspoon, until a pliable dough forms.
4. Separate the dough into 2 large balls. Use a spoon or spatula to spread each ball into a ¼-inch-thick, 8-inch round on the prepared baking sheet.
5. Bake for 15 to 20 minutes, until the center is firm and the edges are browned. Remove from the oven and let cool.
6. These flatbreads can be wrapped up tight and stored in the fridge for up to 4 days. To reheat, bake in a preheated 350°F oven for 8 minutes.

Per Serving

Calories: 395 | Fat: 35.2g | Carbs: 12.4g | Fiber: 7.5g | Protein: 9.3g

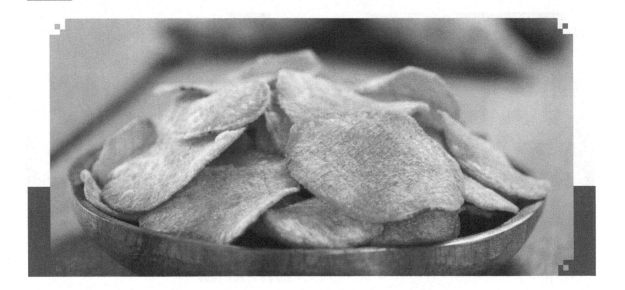

SNICKERDOODLE HAYSTACK COOKIES

Prep time: 5 minutes, plus 30 minutes to chill | Makes 16 cookies | Makes 10 cookies

- ¼ cup (½ stick) unsalted butter, softened
- 2 ounces cream cheese (¼ cup), softened
- ⅓ cup powdered erythritol
- 1 teaspoon ground cinnamon
- ½ teaspoon pure vanilla extract
- ¼ teaspoon baking soda
- 2 cups unsweetened shredded coconut

1. Line a plate or small sheet pan with parchment paper.
2. Place the butter and cream cheese in a medium-sized bowl. Using an electric mixer, beat until smooth.
3. Add the sweetener, cinnamon, vanilla extract, and baking soda and beat for 10 seconds. Stir in the shredded coconut by hand until fully mixed.
4. Use a 1½-tablespoon cookie dough scoop to drop 10 mounded scoops onto the lined plate. Chill for 30 minutes before serving. Store in an airtight container in the refrigerator for up to 1 week or in the freezer for up to 3 months.

Per Serving

Calories: **181** | Fat: **18g** | Protein: **2g** | Carbs: **5g** | Fiber: **3g**

SWEET POTATO CHIPS

Prep time: 20 minutes | Cook time: 2 hours| Serves 8

- 3 large sweet potatoes, sliced as thin as possible
- 3 tablespoons extra-virgin olive oil
- 1 teaspoon sea salt

1. Preheat the oven to 250°F.
2. Position the rack in the center of the oven.
3. In a large bowl, toss the sweet potatoes slices with the olive oil. Arrange the slices in a single layer on two baking sheets. Sprinkle with the sea salt.
4. Place the sheets in the preheated oven and bake for about 2 hours, rotating the pans and flipping the chips after 1 hour.
5. Once the chips are lightly brown and crisp, remove them from the oven. Some may be a bit soft, but they will crisp as they cool.Cool the chips for 10 minutes before serving.
6. Serve immediately. The chips lose their crunch within several hours.

Per Serving

Calories: **267** | Fat: **11g** |Carbs: **42g** |Fiber: **6g** | Protein: **2g**

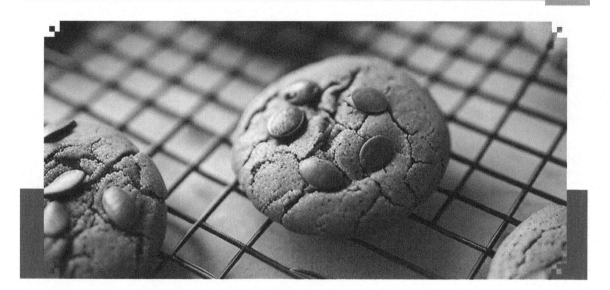

EGG-FREE VANILLA SPICE COOKIES

Prep time: 15 minutes | Cook time: 15 minutes | Makes 10 cookies

- 1½ cups raw pumpkin seeds
- 2 tablespoons coconut flour
- 1 tablespoon flaxseed meal
- 1 tablespoon water
- ⅓ cup granulated erythritol or other low-carb sweetener
- 3 tablespoons coconut oil or lard, softened
- 2 teaspoons pure vanilla extract
- 2 tablespoons unflavored grass-fed beef gelatin (optional)
- 1 teaspoon ground cinnamon
- ½ teaspoon fine Himalayan salt
- ¼ to ½ teaspoon ground cardamom
- ⅓ cup full-fat coconut milk

1. Preheat the oven to 350°F. Line a baking sheet with parchment paper.
2. Combine the pumpkin seeds and coconut flour in a high-powered blender, food processor, or coffee grinder. Process until ground to a fine crumb. Set aside.
3. In a large bowl, combine the flaxseed meal and water and let sit for 2 minutes. Add the erythritol, coconut oil, and vanilla extract and mix until well combined. Add the pumpkin-seed-and-coconut-flour mixture, gelatin (if using), cinnamon, salt, and cardamom. Whisk until a dry dough forms. Add the coconut milk and use a rubber spatula to mix until the dough is moist and uniform.
4. Using a tablespoon, shape 2 tablespoons of the dough into a ball and place it on the prepared baking sheet, then gently flatten. Repeat until all the dough is used, spacing the cookies 2 inches apart. You should get about ten cookies.
5. Bake for 15 minutes, or until the edges are lightly browned. Remove from the oven and let cool to room temperature before handling.
6. Store in an airtight container at room temperature for up to 4 days.

Per Serving

Calories: 193 | Fat: 16.4g | Carbs: 6.6g | Fiber: 2.5g | Protein: 7.2g

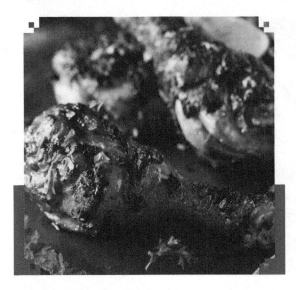

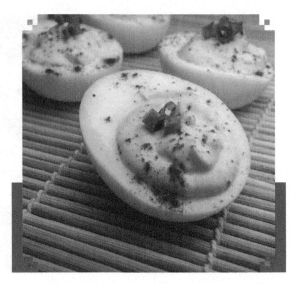

JERK CHICKEN

Prep time: 2 minutes | Cook time: 35 minutes | Serves 8

- 8 whole chicken legs (drumsticks and thighs)
- 3 tablespoons Jerk Seasoning
- 2 teaspoons kosher salt
- 1 cup Easy Keto BBQ Sauce

1. Preheat a grill to medium heat.
2. Coat the chicken legs liberally with the jerk seasoning and salt. Grill the chicken for 20 minutes, turning occasionally.
3. Brush the BBQ sauce on the chicken and grill for 5 more minutes per side, or until a meat thermometer inserted in the thickest part of a thigh reads 165°F.

Per Serving

Calories: 350 | Fat: 20g | Protein: 38g | Carbs: 3g | Fiber: 0.5g

CHIPOTLE DEVILED EGGS

Prep time: 10 minutes, plus time to chill | Cook time: 12 to 15 minutes | Makes 12 deviled eggs

- 6 hard-boiled eggs, peeled
- ¼ cup sugar-free mayonnaise
- 2 tablespoons canned chipotles in adobo sauce
- 1 tablespoon lime juice
- ¼ teaspoon kosher salt

For Garnish (Optional):

- Chipotle powder or paprika
- Chopped fresh parsley

1. Cut the hard-boiled eggs in half lengthwise. Carefully remove the yolks with a spoon and place in a small blender; set the whites aside. Add the mayonnaise, chipotles, lime juice, and salt to the blender and blend for 30 seconds, or until creamy.
2. Transfer the yolk mixture to a resealable plastic bag and cut the tip off of one bottom corner to create a hole about ½ inch in diameter.
3. Squeezing the yolk mixture through the cut-off corner of the bag, pipe about 1 tablespoon of the filling into each egg white half. Sprinkle with chipotle powder or paprika and chopped parsley, if desired. Chill before serving. Store in an airtight container in the refrigerator for up to 5 days.

Per Serving

Calories: 134 | Fat: 12g | Protein: 6g | Carbs: 0.6g | Fiber:0g

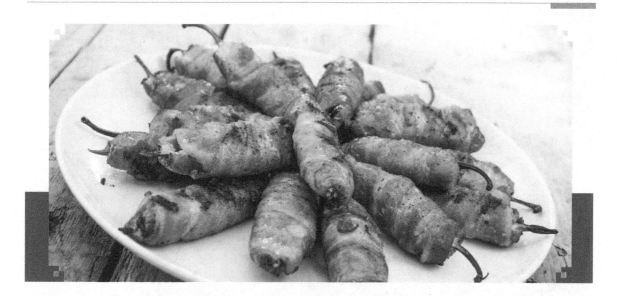

COCONUT PALETAS

Prep time: 6 minutes, plus 3 to 4 hours to chill | Cook time: 15 minutes | Makes 6 paletas

- 1 (14-ounce) can full-fat unsweetened coconut milk
- 3 tablespoons granulated erythritol
- 1 teaspoon pure vanilla extract
- Melted chocolate, chopped almonds, and/ or toasted shredded coconut, for topping (optional)

Special Equipment:

- 6 (3-ounce) ice pop molds

1. Place the coconut milk, sweetener, and vanilla extract in a blender and blend for 30 seconds. Let the mixture rest for 5 minutes, then stir gently until any foam at the top has disappeared. Pour into 6 ice pop molds and freeze until firm, 3 to 4 hours. Store in the freezer until ready to eat.
2. Before serving, unmold the ice pops and sprinkle with chopped almonds or toasted coconut and drizzle with melted chocolate, if desired. Store in the freezer for up to 1 month.

Per Serving

Calories: **100** | Fat: **10g** | Protein:**0g** | Carbs: **1g** | Fiber:**0g**

BACON-WRAPPED JALAPEÑOS

Prep time: 10 minutes | Cook time: 20 minutes | Serves 4

- 10 jalapeños
- 8 ounces cream cheese, at room temperature
- 1 pound bacon (you will use about half a slice per popper)

1. Preheat the oven to 450°F. Line a baking sheet with aluminum foil or a silicone baking mat.
2. Halve the jalapeños lengthwise, and remove the seeds and membranes (if you like the extra heat, leave them in). Place them on the prepared pan cut-side up.
3. Spread some of the cream cheese inside each jalapeño half.
4. Wrap a jalapeño half with a slice of bacon (depending on the size of the jalapeño, use a whole slice of bacon, or half).
5. Secure the bacon around each jalapeño with 1 to 2 toothpicks so it stays put while baking.
6. Bake for 20 minutes, until the bacon is done and crispy.
7. Serve hot or at room temperature. Either way, they are delicious!

Per Serving

Calories: **164** | Fat: **13g** | Carbs: **1g** | Fiber: **0g** | Protein: **9g**

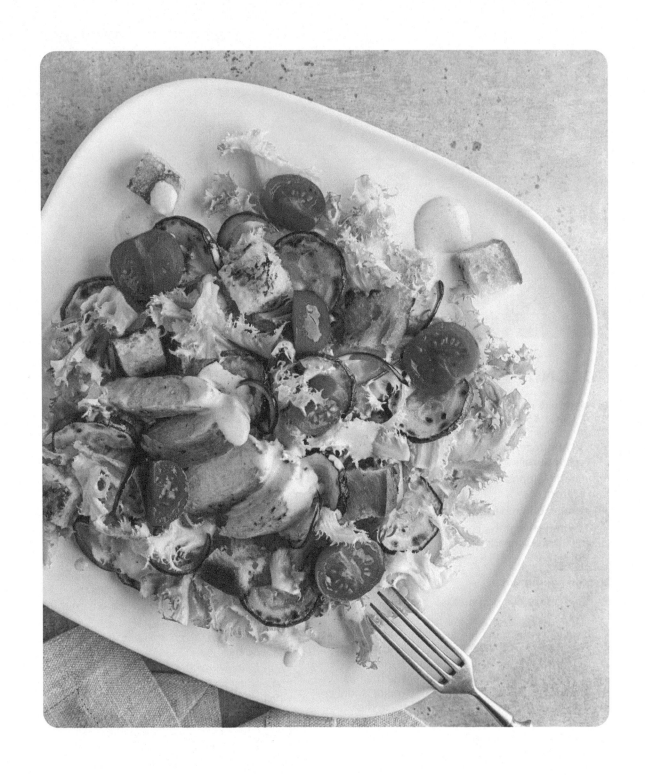

CHAPTER 5: POULTRY

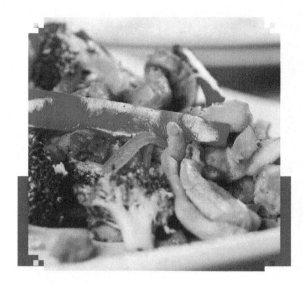

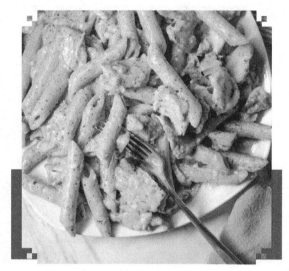

CHICKEN STIR-FRY

Prep time: **15 minutes** | Cook time: **15 minutes** | Serves **4**

- 3 tablespoons extra-virgin olive oil
- 6 scallions, white and green parts, chopped
- 1 cup broccoli florets
- 1 pound boneless, skinless chicken breasts, cut into bite-size pieces
- 1 recipe stir-fry sauce
- Tablespoons toasted sesame seeds (optional)

1. In a large nonstick skillet over medium-high heat, heat the olive oil until it shimmers.
2. Add the scallions, broccoli, and chicken. Cook for 5 to 7 minutes, stirring occasionally, until the chicken is cooked and the vegetables are tender.
3. Add the stir-fry sauce. Cook for 5 minutes, stirring, until the sauce reduces.
4. Garnish with sesame seeds, if using.

Per Serving

Calories: **363** | Fat: **22g** |Carbs: **7g** | Fiber: **2g** | Protein: **36g**

CREAMY CHICKEN PESTO PASTA

Prep time: **10 minutes** | Cook time: **10 minutes** | Serves **6**

- 3 cups brown rice fusilli
- 1 cup diced cooked chicken breast
- 1 cup Pistachio Pesto
- 1 cup plain whole-milk Greek yogurt
- 1 red bell pepper, diced
- 1 tablespoon minced shallot
- 2 teaspoons freshly squeezed lemon juice
- ½ teaspoon salt
- ¼ teaspoon freshly ground black pepper

1. Cook the pasta according to the package instructions and drain. Transfer to a large bowl.
2. Add the chicken, pistachio pesto, yogurt, red bell pepper, shallot, lemon juice, salt, and pepper. Stir well.
3. Serve chilled, if desired.

Per Serving

Calories: **286** | Fat: **12g** | Carbs: **26g** | Fiber: **2g**; | Protein: **20g**

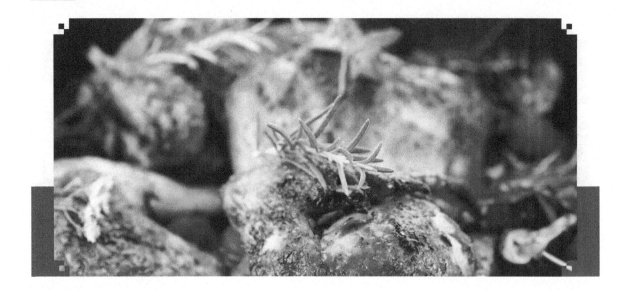

SALSA VERDE CHICKEN

Prep time: **15 minutes** | Cook time: **6 to 8 hours** | Serves **6**

*   4 to 5 boneless, skinless chicken breasts (about 2 pounds)
*   2 cups green salsa
*   1 cup chicken broth
*   2 tablespoons freshly squeezed lime juice
*   1 teaspoon sea salt
*   1 teaspoon chili powder

1. In your slow cooker, combine the chicken, salsa, broth, lime juice, salt, and chili powder. Stir to combine.
2. Cover the cooker and set to low. Cook for 6 to 8 hours, or until the internal temperature of the chicken reaches 165°F on a meat thermometer and the juices run clear.
3. Shred the chicken with a fork, mix it into the sauce, and serve.

Per Serving

Calories: **318** | Fat: **8g** | Carbs: **6g** | Fiber: **1g** | Protein: **52g**

HERB-ROASTED CHICKEN

Prep time: **15 minutes** | Cook time: **1 hour, 30 minutes** | Serves **4**

*   1 (4-pound) whole chicken, rinsed and patted dry
*   2 lemons, halved
*   1 sweet onion, quartered
*   4 garlic cloves, crushed
*   6 fresh thyme sprigs
*   6 fresh rosemary sprigs
*   3 bay leaves
*   2 tablespoons olive oil
*   Sea salt
*   Freshly ground black pepper

1. Preheat the oven to 400°F.
2. Place the chicken in a roasting pan. Stuff the lemons, onion, garlic, thyme, rosemary, and bay leaves into the cavity. Brush the chicken with the olive oil, and season lightly with sea salt and pepper.
3. Roast the chicken for about 1½ hours until golden brown and cooked through.
4. Remove the chicken from the oven and let it sit for 10 minutes. Remove the lemons, onion, and herbs from the cavity and serve.

Per Serving

Calories: **261** | Fat: **9g** | Carbs: **5g** | Fiber: **2g** | Protein: **38g**

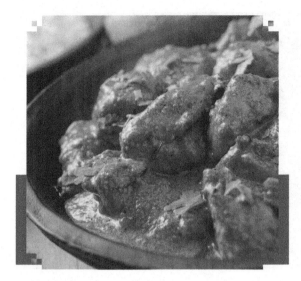

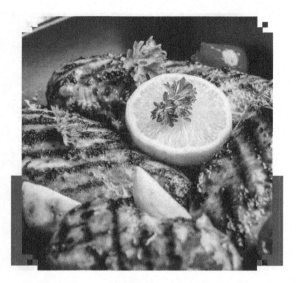

GREEN CHICKEN CURRY

Prep time: 5 minutes | Cook time: 12 minutes | Serves 4

- 3 tablespoons green curry paste
- 1 tablespoon coconut oil
- 1 (14-ounce) can full-fat unsweetened coconut milk
- 3 tablespoons granulated erythritol
- 2 tablespoons fish sauce (no sugar added)
- 2 cups broccoli florets
- 1 pound boneless, skinless chicken breasts, cut into thin strips
- ½ cup sliced yellow bell peppers
- ½ cup sliced bamboo shoots, drained
- 1 tablespoon sliced chili peppers
- Fresh cilantro leaves, for garnish

1. Combine the curry paste and coconut oil in a large skillet and cook over medium heat for 2 minutes, or until fragrant.
2. Whisk in the coconut milk, sweetener, and fish sauce until smooth. Add the broccoli and simmer over medium-low heat for 5 minutes, being careful not to allow the mixture to boil.
3. Add the chicken, bell peppers, bamboo shoots, and chili peppers. Simmer, stirring occasionally, for another 5 minutes, or until the chicken is cooked through and the broccoli is fork-tender. Garnish with cilantro and serve hot.

Per Serving

Calories: **301** | Fat: **20g** | Protein: **29g** | Carbs: **8g** | Fiber: **4g**

MEDITERRANEAN CHICKEN BAKE

Prep time: 10 minutes | Cook time: 20 minutes | Serves 4

- 4 (4-ounce) boneless, skinless chicken breasts
- 2 tablespoons avocado oil
- 1 pint cherry tomatoes, halved
- 1 cup packed chopped fresh spinach
- 1 cup sliced cremini mushrooms
- ½ red onion, thinly sliced
- ½ cup chopped fresh basil
- 4 garlic cloves, minced
- 2 teaspoons balsamic vinegar

1. Preheat the oven to 400°F.
2. Place the chicken breasts in a glass baking dish. Brush with the avocado oil.
3. In a medium bowl, stir together the tomatoes, spinach, mushrooms, red onion, basil, garlic, and vinegar.
4. Top each chicken breast with one-fourth of the vegetable mixture.
5. Bake for about 20 minutes, or until the chicken is cooked through.

Per Serving

Calories: **219** | Fat: **9g** | Carbs: **7g** | Fiber: **2g;** | Protein: **28g**

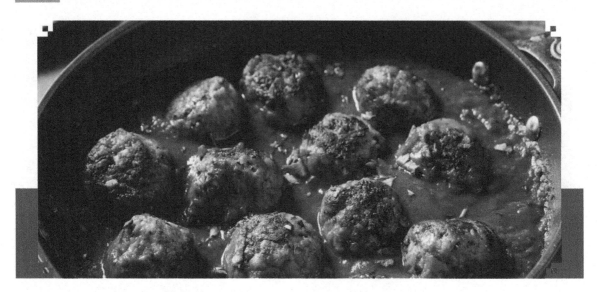

TURKEY SLOPPY JOES

Prep time: **15 minutes** | Cook time: **4 to 6 hours** | Serves **6**

- 1 tablespoon extra-virgin olive oil
- 1 pound ground turkey
- 1 celery stalk, minced
- 1 carrot, minced
- ½ medium sweet onion, diced
- ½ red bell pepper, finely chopped
- 6 tablespoons tomato paste
- 2 tablespoons apple cider vinegar
- 1 tablespoon maple syrup
- 1 teaspoon Dijon mustard
- 1 teaspoon chili powder
- ½ teaspoon garlic powder
- ½ teaspoon sea salt
- ½ teaspoon dried oregano

1. In your slow cooker, combine the olive oil, turkey, celery, carrot, onion, red bell pepper, tomato paste, vinegar, maple syrup, mustard, chili powder, garlic powder, salt, and oregano. Using a large spoon, break up the turkey into smaller chunks as it combines with the other ingredients.
2. Cover the cooker and set to low. Cook for 4 to 6 hours, stir thoroughly, and serve.

Per Serving

Calories: **251** | Fat: **12g** | Carbs: **14g** | Fiber: **3g** | Protein: **24g**

GINGERED TURKEY MEATBALLS

Prep time: **10 minutes** | Cook time: **10 minutes** | Serves **4**

- 1½ pounds ground turkey
- 1 cup shredded cabbage
- ¼ cup chopped fresh cilantro leaves
- 1 tablespoon grated fresh ginger
- 1 teaspoon garlic powder
- 1 teaspoon onion powder
- ½ teaspoon sea salt
- ⅛ teaspoon freshly ground black pepper
- 2 tablespoons olive oil

1. In a large bowl, combine the turkey, cabbage, cilantro, ginger, garlic powder, onion powder, salt, and pepper. Mix well. Form the turkey mixture into about 20 (¾-inch) meatballs.
2. In a large nonstick skillet over medium-high heat, heat the olive oil until it shimmers.
3. Add the meatballs and cook for about 10 minutes, turning as they brown.

Per Serving

Calories: **408** | Fat: **26g** | Carbs: **4g** | Fiber: **1g** | Protein: **47g**

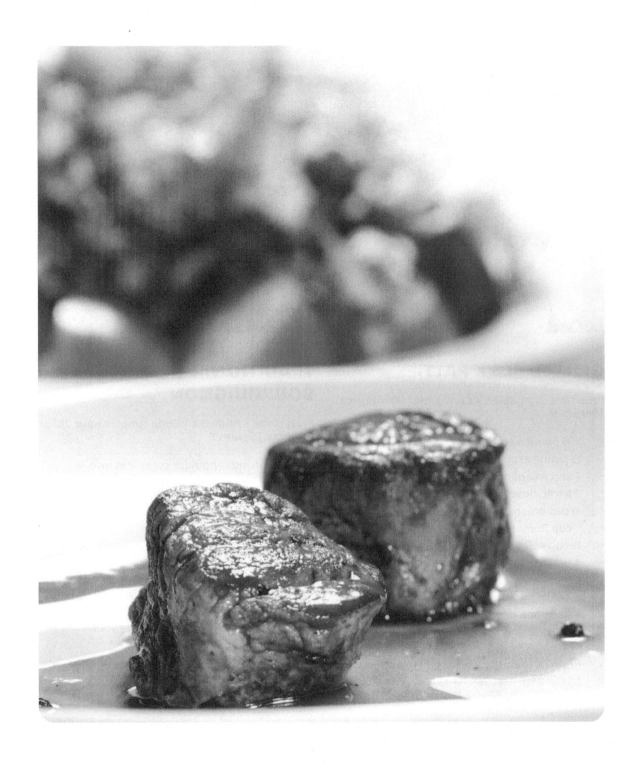

CHAPTER 6: PORK, BEEF AND LAMB

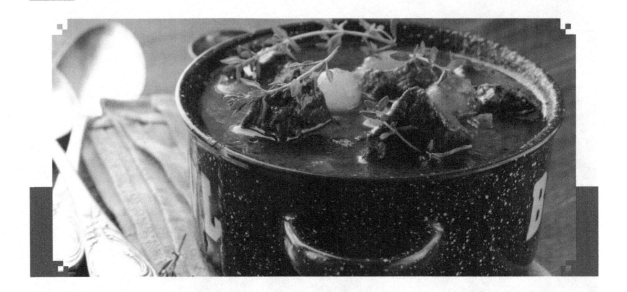

GRILLED PORK PATTIES

Prep time: 5 minutes | Cook time: 20 minutes | Serves 6

- 1 ½ pounds ground pork
- ½ pound ground turkey
- 1 serrano pepper, deseeded and minced
- 2 garlic cloves, finely minced
- ½ cup onion, finely minced
- 1 cup Romano cheese, grated
- ½ cup Asiago cheese, shredded
- 1 teaspoon mustard seeds
- ½ teaspoon dried marjoram
- ½ teaspoon dried basil
- 1 teaspoon paprika
- Sea salt and ground black pepper, to taste

1. Begin by preheating a gas grill to high.
2. Mix all of the above ingredients until everything is well incorporated. Form the mixture into 6 patties with oiled hands.
3. Place on the preheated grill and cook for 7 to 8 minutes on each side until slightly charred. Bon appétit!

Per Serving

Calories: 515 | Fat: 35.4g | Carbs:2.6g | Protein: 44.3g | Fiber: 0.2g

TRADITIONAL BEEF BOURGUIGNON

Prep time: 5 minutes | Cook time: 1 hour 20 minutes | Serves 5

- 1 ½ pounds shoulder steak, cut into cubes
- 1 tablespoon Herbs de Provence
- 1 onion, chopped
- 1 celery stalk, chopped
- 1 cup red Burgundy wine

1. Heat up a lightly greased soup pot over a medium-high flame. Now brown the beef in batches until no longer pink.
2. Add a splash of wine to deglaze your pan.
3. Add the Herbs de Provence, onion, celery, and wine to the pot; pour in 3 cups of water and stir to combine well. Bring to a rapid boil; then, turn the heat to medium-low.
4. Cover and let it simmer for 1 hour 10 minutes. Serve over hot cauliflower rice if desired.
5. Enjoy!

Per Serving

Calories: 217 | Fat: 5.5g | Carbs: 3.9g | Protein: 30g | Fiber: 0.4g

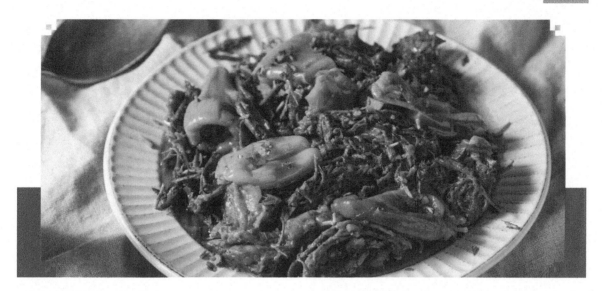

MISSISSIPPI POT ROAST

Prep time: **5 minutes** | Cook time: **8 hours** | Serves **4**

- 1 pound beef chuck roast
- Pink Himalayan salt
- Freshly ground black pepper
- 1 (1-ounce) packet dry Au Jus Gravy Mix
- 1 (1-ounce) packet dry ranch dressing
- 8 tablespoons butter (1 stick)
- 1 cup whole pepperoncini (I use Mezzetta)

1. with the crock insert in place, preheat the slow cooker to low.
2. Season both sides of the beef chuck roast with pink Himalayan salt and pepper. Put in the slow cooker.
3. Sprinkle the gravy mix and ranch dressing packets on top of the roast.
4. Place the butter on top of the roast, and sprinkle the pepperoncini around it.
5. Cover and cook on low for 8 hours.
6. Shred the beef using two forks, and serve hot.

Per Serving

Calories: **504** | Fat: **34g** | Carbs: **6g** |Fiber: **0g** | Protein: **36g**

BEEF SAUSAGE MEAT LOAF

Prep time: **10 minutes** | Cook time: **1 Hour and 15 minutes** | Serves **6**

- 1½ pounds Italian sausage meat
- 1 pound grass-fed ground beef
- ½ cup almond flour
- ¼ cup heavy (whipping) cream
- 1 egg, lightly beaten
- ½ onion, finely chopped
- ½ red bell pepper, chopped
- 2 teaspoons minced garlic
- 1 teaspoon dried oregano
- ¼ teaspoon sea salt
- ⅛ teaspoon freshly ground black pepper

1. Preheat the oven. Set the oven temperature to 400°F.
2. Make the meat loaf. In a large bowl, mix together the sausage, ground beef, almond flour, cream, egg, onion, red bell pepper, garlic, oregano, salt, and pepper until everything is well combined. Press the mixture into a 9-inch loaf pan.
3. Bake. Bake for 1 hour to 1 hour and 15 minutes, or until the meat loaf is cooked through. Drain off and throw out any grease and let the meat loaf stand for 10 minutes.
4. Serve. Cut the meat loaf into six slices, divide them between six plates, and serve it immediately.

Per Serving

Calories: **394** | Fat: **34g** | Carbs: **1g** | Fiber: **0g** | Protein: **19g**

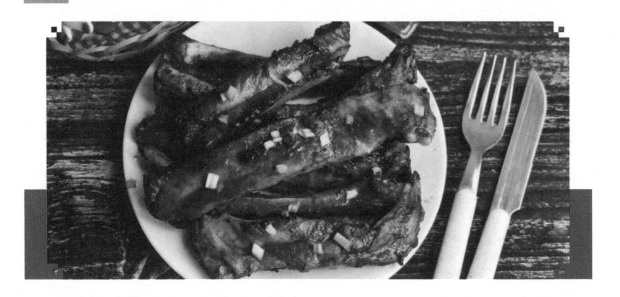

SALT AND PEPPER RIBS

Prep time: **10 minutes** | Cook time: **35 minutes** | Serves 8

- 3⅓ pounds country-style pork ribs
- 2 cups chicken bone broth, or more as needed
- 1 tablespoon finely ground gray sea salt
- 2 teaspoons ground black pepper
- 1 batch Kickin' Ketchup, for serving (optional)

1. Stand the ribs up around the inside wall of a pressure cooker or slow cooker, keeping the same side of the ribs facing outward. Add enough broth to come halfway up the sides of the ribs.
2. If using a pressure cooker, seal the lid and cook on high pressure for 15 minutes (for riblets) or 25 minutes (for full side ribs). If using a slow cooker, cook on low for 4 hours or on high for 2 hours. The ribs are perfectly cooked when the meat is tender but is still firmly attached to the bone; make sure to remove the ribs before the meat falls off the bones.
3. Transfer the cooked ribs and cooking liquid to a shallow baking dish. Once cool, cover and refrigerate overnight.
4. When ready to cook the ribs, preheat a grill to medium heat (350°F/177°C) or, if using the oven, place an oven rack in the top position and preheat the oven to 400°F (205°C).
5. Remove the ribs from the fridge. There will be hardened fats all around them. Slather the fats on the meaty top of each rib. Coat the ribs all over in the salt and pepper.
6. If finishing the ribs in the oven, place them on an unlined rimmed baking sheet and cook for 10 minutes, just until heated through. Then turn the broiler to low if that is an option; otherwise, simply "broil" is fine. Broil for 5 to 7 minutes, just until crisp. If finishing the ribs on the grill, place the ribs in the preheated grill and cook for 1 to 2 minutes per side to heat them up and give them a crispy exterior.
7. Transfer to a serving plate and dig in!

Per Serving

Calories: **374** | Fat: **26.5g** | Carbs: **0.5g** | Fiber: **0g** | Protein: **33.3g**

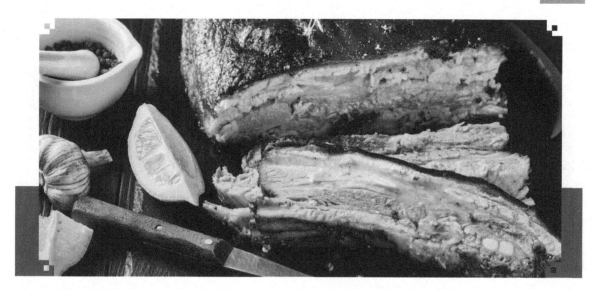

CILANTRO GARLIC PORK CHOPS

Prep time: 10 minutes | Cook time: 15 minutes | Serves 4

- 1 pound boneless center-cut pork chops, pounded to ¼ inch thick
- Sea salt, for seasoning
- Freshly ground black pepper, for seasoning
- ¼ cup good-quality olive oil, divided
- ¼ cup finely chopped fresh cilantro
- 1 tablespoon minced garlic
- Juice of 1 lime

1. Marinate the pork. Pat the pork chops dry and season them lightly with salt and pepper. Place them in a large bowl, add 2 tablespoons of the olive oil, and the cilantro, garlic, and lime juice. Toss to coat the chops. Cover the bowl and marinate the chops at room temperature for 30 minutes.
2. Cook the pork. In a large skillet over medium-high heat, warm the remaining 2 tablespoons of olive oil. Add the pork chops in a single layer and fry them, turning them once, until they're just cooked through and still juicy, 6 to 7 minutes per side.
3. Serve. Divide the chops between four plates and serve them immediately.

Per Serving

Calories: **249** | Fat: **16g** | Carbs: **2g** | Fiber: **0g** | Protein: **25g**

EASY JERK RIBS

Prep time: 2 minutes | Cook time: 1 hour 45 minutes | Serves 4

- 1 rack baby back ribs
- ¼ cup Jerk Seasoning
- 2 teaspoons kosher salt
- ½ cup Easy Keto BBQ Sauce

1. Preheat a grill to medium heat. Generously season the rack of ribs on both sides with the jerk seasoning and salt. Grill for 15 minutes per side over direct heat. The ribs should be browned and crispy looking on the outside.
2. Wrap the ribs loosely in foil and place on the grill over indirect heat. You may need to move coals to the side, or turn off one or two burners to create a flame-free space. with the lid closed, cook the ribs for 1 hour; the grill temperature should be about 350°F.
3. After 1 hour, open the foil and baste the ribs on both sides with the BBQ sauce. Cook for 30 more minutes, or until the ribs are done to your desired tenderness. Cut into individual ribs to serve.

Per Serving

Calories: **390** | Fat: **27g** | Protein: **26g** | Carbs: **6g** | Fiber: **2g**

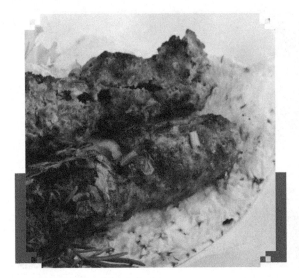

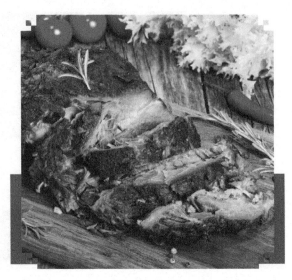

GRILLED HERBED PORK KEBABS

Prep time: **10 minutes** | Cook time: **15 minutes** | Serves **4**

- ¼ cup good-quality olive oil
- 1 tablespoon minced garlic
- 2 teaspoons dried oregano
- 1 teaspoon dried basil
- 1 teaspoon dried
- parsley
- ½ teaspoon sea salt
- ¼ teaspoon freshly ground black pepper
- 1 (1-pound) pork tenderloin, cut into 1½-inch pieces

1. Marinate the pork. In a medium bowl, stir together the olive oil, garlic, oregano, basil, parsley, salt, and pepper. Add the pork pieces and toss to coat them in the marinade. Cover the bowl and place it in the refrigerator for 2 to 4 hours.
2. Make the kebabs. Divide the pork pieces between four skewers, making sure to not crowd the meat.
3. Grill the kebabs. Preheat your grill to medium-high heat. Grill the skewers for about 12 minutes, turning to cook all sides of the pork, until the pork is cooked through.
4. Serve. Rest the skewers for 5 minutes. Divide the skewers between four plates and serve them immediately.

Per Serving

Calories: **261** | Fat: **18g** | Carbs: **1g** | Fiber: **0g** | Protein: **24g**

ITALIAN PORK ROAST WITH PEPPERS

Prep time: **5 minutes** | Cook time: **20 minutes** | Serves **6**

- 2 tablespoons olive oil
- 2 pounds pork roast, sliced
- ¼ cup red wine
- 2 Italian peppers, chopped
- 2 scallions, chopped
- 2 garlic cloves, minced
- Sea salt and ground black pepper, to season
- 2 teaspoons Italian seasoning mix
- ½ cup vegetable broth

1. Heat the olive oil in a saucepan over a moderate flame. Once hot, sear the pork roast for 3 to 4 minutes per side; reserve.
2. Add a splash of wine to deglaze the pan.
3. Add in the Italian peppers and continue to sauté for 3 minutes more or until they are tender; add in the scallions and garlic and continue to sauté a minute more or until aromatic.
4. Sprinkle with salt, black pepper, and Italian seasoning mix. Pour in the vegetable broth and any remaining wine.
5. Add the pork back to the pan. Let it cook, covered, over medium-low heat for 10 minutes more until heated through. Bon appétit!

Per Serving

Calories: **255** | Fat: **10.9g** | Carbs: **3.4g** | Protein: **24.4g** | Fiber: **0.6g**

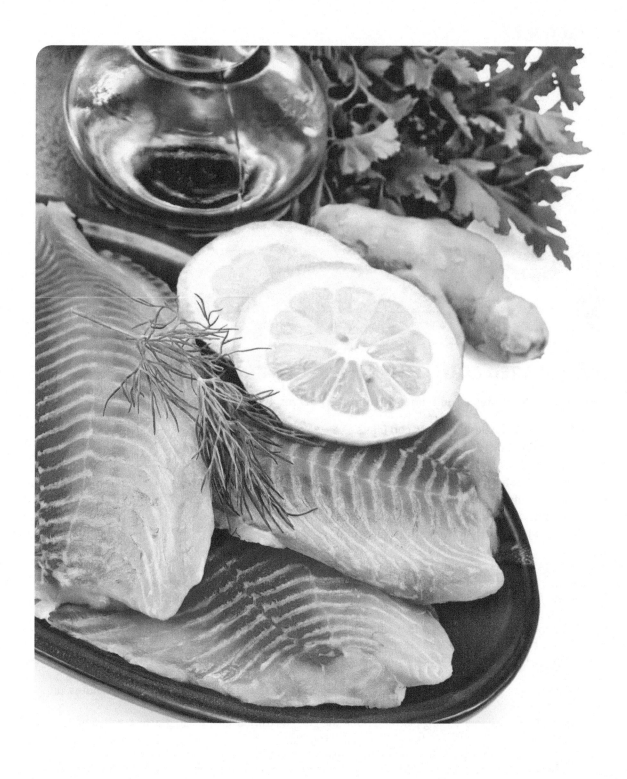

CHAPTER 7: FISH AND SEAFOOD

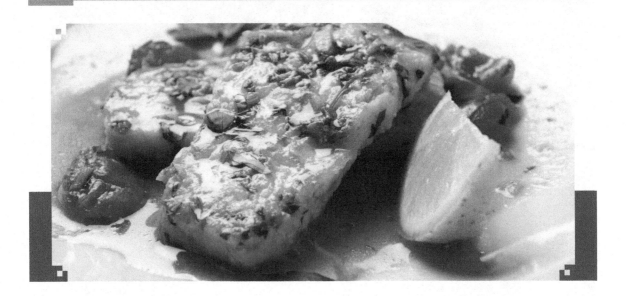

PAN-SEARED COD

Prep time: 10 minutes | Cook time: 10 minutes | Serves 4

- 4 (6-ounce) boneless, skinless cod fillets
- 1 teaspoon fine Himalayan salt
- 3 tablespoons ghee or bacon fat
- 2 sprigs fresh parsley
- 1 green onion, sliced
- 1 tablespoon Garlic Confit
- Lime or lemon halves, for garnish (optional)

1. Pat the fish fillets dry and rub the salt all over them.
2. Heat a large cast-iron skillet over medium heat until it's very hot, rotating the pan halfway every few minutes. Drip water on it to check the temperature; when the droplets dance, it's ready.
3. Melt the ghee in the skillet. Add the fish fillets, being careful not to crowd the pan—cook two fillets at a time if you have to. Sear the fish for 4 to 6 minutes. When the edges of the fish begin to look opaque white and you can see that it is golden underneath, use a thin spatula to flip the fish.
4. Place the parsley, green onion slices, and garlic confit around the fish. Cook for 3 to 4 minutes, until the fish is tender and flakes easily with a fork.
5. Transfer the fish to a serving platter. Spoon the ghee mixture over the fish. Garnish with lime halves, if desired. Let it rest for 3 to 5 minutes before serving.
6. I'm not a fan of leftover fish. Cook as many fillets as you have people to feed to avoid having leftovers. If they can't be avoided, store leftovers in an airtight container in the fridge for up to 3 days.

Per Serving

Calories: 223 | Fat: 11.3g | Carbs: 2.5g | Fiber: 0.1g | Protein: 27.5g

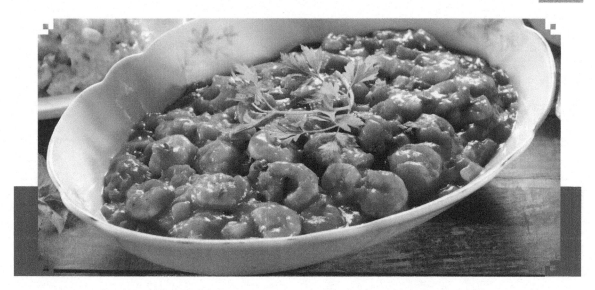

WHITEFISH WITH SPICE RUB

Prep time: 3 minutes | Cook time: 12 minutes | Serves 4

- 2 tablespoons Slow-Cooker Ghee, melted, divided
- 4 (6-ounce) whitefish fillets
- 1 tablespoon paprika
- 2 teaspoons ground cumin
- 2 teaspoons onion powder
- 2 teaspoons salt
- 1 teaspoon ground turmeric
- ½ teaspoon freshly ground black pepper
- 1 tablespoon coconut sugar (optional)

1. Preheat the oven to 400°F.
2. Brush a shallow baking dish with 1 tablespoon of ghee.
3. Place the fish fillets in the dish and brush them with the remaining 1 tablespoon of ghee.
4. In a small bowl, combine the paprika, cumin, onion powder, salt, turmeric, pepper, and coconut sugar (if using).
5. Use 1 tablespoon of the spice rub on the fillets, making sure the surface of the fish is covered with rub. Store the remaining rub for future use.
6. Place the baking dish in the preheated oven and bake the fish for 12 to 15 minutes, or until firm and cooked through.

Per Serving

Calories: **364** | Fat: **20g** | Carbs: **3g** | Fiber: **1g** | Protein: **42g**

SHRIMP WITH CINNAMON SAUCE

Prep time: 10 minutes | Cook time: 10 minutes | Serves 4

- 2 tablespoons extra-virgin olive oil
- 1½ pounds peeled shrimp
- 2 tablespoons dijon mustard
- 1 cup no-salt-added chicken broth
- 1 teaspoon ground cinnamon
- 1 teaspoon onion powder
- ½ teaspoon sea salt
- ¼ teaspoon freshly ground black pepper

1. In a large nonstick skillet over medium-high heat, heat the olive oil until it shimmers.
2. Add the shrimp. Cook for about 4 minutes, stirring occasionally, until the shrimp is opaque.
3. In a small bowl, whisk the mustard, chicken broth, cinnamon, onion powder, salt, and pepper. Pour this into the skillet and continue to cook for 3 minutes, stirring occasionally.

Per Serving

Calories: **270** | Fat: **11g** | Carbs: **4g** | Fiber: **1g** | Protein: **39g**

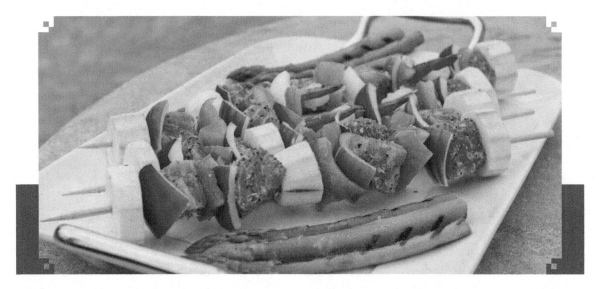

OPEN-FACE AVOCADO TUNA MELTS

Prep time: **10 minutes** | Cook time: **5 minutes** | Serves **4**

- 4 slices sourdough bread
- 2 (5-ounce) cans wild-caught albacore tuna
- ¼ cup Paleo mayonnaise
- 2 tablespoons minced shallot
- 1 teaspoon freshly squeezed lemon juice
- Dash garlic powder
- Dash paprika
- 1 large avocado, cut in 8 slices
- 1 large tomato, cut in 8 slices
- ¼ cup shredded raw Parmesan cheese, divided

1. Preheat the broiler.
2. Line a baking sheet with aluminum foil.
3. Arrange the slices of bread in the prepared pan.
4. In a medium bowl, mix the tuna, mayonnaise, shallot, lemon juice, garlic powder, and paprika. Spread one-fourth of the tuna mixture on each slice of bread.
5. Top each with 2 of the avocado slices and 2 of the tomato slices.
6. Sprinkle each with 1 tablespoon of Parmesan cheese.
7. Broil for 3 to 4 minutes, watching carefully so they don't burn. Serve hot.

Per Serving

Calories: **471** | Fat: **27g** | Carbs: **31g** | Fiber: **4g;** | Protein: **27g**

SALMON & ASPARAGUS SKEWERS

Prep time: **15 minutes** | Cook time: **10 minutes** | Serves **8**

- 2 tablespoons ghee, melted
- 1 teaspoon Dijon mustard
- 1 teaspoon garlic powder
- ½ teaspoon salt
- ¼ teaspoon red pepper flakes
- 1½ pounds boned skinless salmon, cut into 2-inch chunks
- 2 lemons, thinly sliced
- 1 bunch asparagus spears, tough ends trimmed, cut into 2-inch pieces

1. Preheat the broiler.
2. Line a baking sheet with aluminum foil.
3. In a small saucepan over medium heat, heat the ghee.
4. Stir in the mustard, garlic powder, salt, and red pepper flakes.
5. On each skewer, thread 1 chunk of salmon, 1 lemon slice folded in half, and 2 pieces of asparagus. Repeat with the remaining skewers until all ingredients are used. Place the skewers on the prepared pan and brush each with the ghee-seasoning mixture.
6. Broil for 4 minutes. Turn the skewers and broil on the other side for about 4 minutes.

Per Serving

Calories: **250** | Fat: **9g** | Carbs: **4g** | Fiber: **2g;** | Protein: **38g**

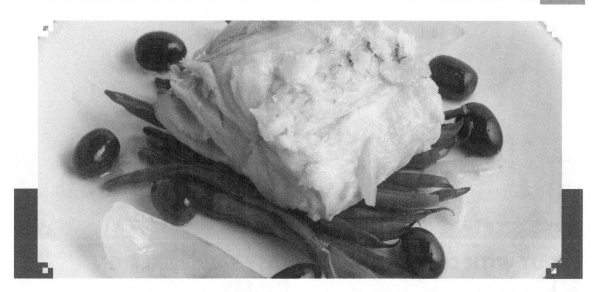

SMOKED SALMON STACKS

Prep time: 15 minutes | **Cook time: 15 minutes** | **Serves 4**

- 8 ounces cold-smoked salmon (lox style)
- 1 cup diced cucumbers
- 1 tablespoon minced red onions
- 1 teaspoon granulated erythritol
- 1 teaspoon white vinegar
- 1 to 2 large ripe Hass avocados, halved and pitted
- 8 cups spring greens
- 8 tablespoons Creamy Lemon Caper Dressing

1. Chop the salmon into ½-inch pieces.
2. Combine the cucumbers, onions, sweetener, and vinegar in a small bowl.
3. Remove the flesh from the avocados and chop into ½-inch pieces.
4. Assemble the stacks: Spread out 2 cups of spring greens on a salad plate. Pack one-quarter of the chopped salmon into a 4-inch ramekin or dish. Top the salmon with one-quarter of the cucumber-onion mixture, then one-quarter of the chopped avocados.
5. Press the stack down gently to compact the layers but do not mash them out of shape. Carefully turn the ramekin over on the salad greens to unmold the stack.
6. Repeat Step 4 until you have four complete stacks. Drizzle 2 tablespoons of the dressing over each stack and serve.

Per Serving

Calories: **248** | Fat: **21g** | Protein: **12g** | Carbs: **5g** | Fiber: **3g**

COD WITH GINGER AND BLACK BEANS

Prep time: 10 minutes | **Cook time: 15 minutes** | **Serves 4**

- 2 tablespoons extra-virgin olive oil
- 4 (6-ounce) cod fillets
- 1 tablespoon grated fresh ginger
- 1 teaspoon sea salt, divided
- ¼ teaspoon freshly ground black pepper
- 5 garlic cloves, minced
- 1 (14-ounce) can black beans, drained
- ¼ cup chopped fresh cilantro leaves

1. In a large nonstick skillet over medium-high heat, heat the olive oil until it shimmers.
2. Season the cod with the ginger, ½ teaspoon of the salt, and the pepper. Place it in the hot oil and cook for about 4 minutes per side until the fish is opaque. Remove the cod from the pan and set it aside on a platter, tented with aluminum foil.
3. Return the skillet to the heat and add the garlic. Cook for 30 seconds, stirring constantly.
4. Stir in the black beans and the remaining ½ teaspoon of salt. Cook for 5 minutes, stirring occasionally.
5. Stir in the cilantro and spoon the black beans over the cod.

Per Serving

Calories: **419** | Fat: **2g** | Carbs: **33g** | Fiber: **8g** | Protein: **50g**

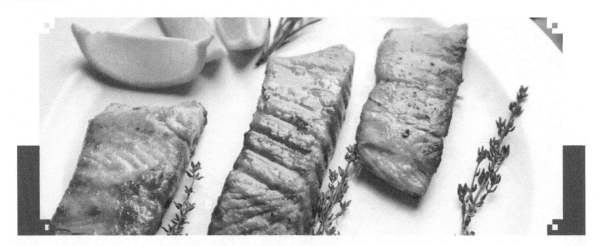

TROUT WITH CUCUMBER SALSA

Prep time: 20 minutes | **Cook time: 10 minutes** | **Serves 4**

For The Salsa:

- 1 English cucumber, diced
- ¼ cup unsweetened coconut yogurt
- 1 scallion, white and green parts,

- chopped
- 2 tablespoons chopped fresh mint
- 1 teaspoon raw honey
- Sea salt

For The Fish:

- 1 tablespoon olive oil
- 4 (5-ounce) trout fillets, patted dry

- Sea salt
- Freshly ground black pepper

To Make The Salsa:

1. In a small bowl, stir together the cucumber, yogurt, scallion, mint, and honey until well mixed. Season with sea salt and set it aside.

To Make The Fish:

1. Place a large skillet over medium heat and add the olive oil.
2. Season the trout lightly with sea salt and pepper. Add it to the skillet and panfry for about 5 minutes per side, turning once, or until it is just cooked through.
3. Top with the cucumber salsa and serve.

Per Serving

Calories: 329 | **Fat: 16g** | **Carbs: 6g** | **Fiber: 1g** | **Protein: 39g**

EASY SAUCY SALMON FILLETS

Prep time: 5 minutes | **Cook time: 20 minutes** |**Serves 6**

- 2 tablespoons peanut oil
- 2 bell peppers, deseeded and sliced
- ½ cup scallions, chopped
- 2 cloves garlic, minced
- 4 tablespoons Marsala wine
- 2 ripe tomatoes, pureed
- 2 ½ pounds salmon fillets
- Sea salt and ground black pepper, to taste
- ¼ teaspoon ground bay leaf
- 1 teaspoon paprika

1. Heat the peanut oil in a large frying pan over a moderate flame. Now, sauté the bell peppers and scallions for 3 minutes.
2. Add in the garlic and continue to sauté for 30 seconds more or until aromatic but not until it's browned.
3. Add a splash of wine to deglaze the pan. Stir in the remaining ingredients and turn the heat to simmer.
4. Let it cook, partially covered, for 15 minutes or until the salmon is cooked through. Bon appétit!

Per Serving

Calories: 347 | **Fat: 18.5g** | **Carbs: 4g** | **Protein: 39.9g** | **Fiber: 1g**

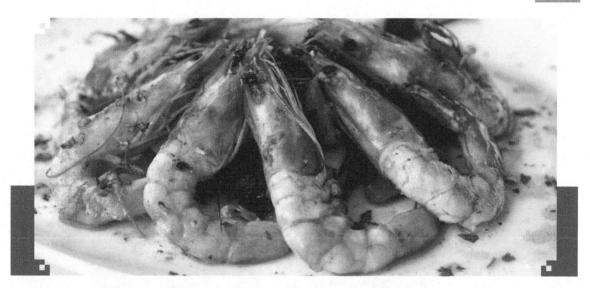

CURRIED POACHED HALIBUT

Prep time: **5 minutes** | Cook time: **23 minutes** | Serves **4**

- 1 tablespoon avocado oil
- ½ cup diced white onion
- 2 garlic cloves, minced
- 1 tablespoon red curry paste
- 1½ cups chicken broth
- 1 (14-ounce) can coconut milk
- ½ teaspoon coconut sugar
- 1 teaspoon salt
- ½ teaspoon freshly ground black pepper
- 4 (4-ounce) halibut fillets

1. In a large skillet over medium heat, heat the avocado oil.
2. Add the onion and garlic, and sauté for 2 to 3 minutes until the onions are translucent.
3. Stir in the curry paste until incorporated.
4. Add the broth, coconut milk, coconut sugar, salt, and pepper and stir to combine. Reduce the heat to medium-low and gently simmer for 10 minutes.
5. Pat the halibut dry with a paper towel. Place each fillet into the curried broth. Cover and poach for 10 minutes. Check the fish for doneness; if it flakes, it should be done. To speed the cooking time, occasionally spoon some broth over the halibut as it cooks.
6. Serve the fillets in four bowls with the curried broth spooned on top.

Per Serving

Calories: **358** | Fat: **22g** | Carbs: **10g** | Fiber: **1g;** | Protein: **28g**

HOT AND SPICY TIGER PRAWNS

Prep time: **5 minutes** | Cook time: **15 minutes** | Serves **6**

- 2 tablespoons olive oil
- 1 teaspoon ghee
- 2 scallions, chopped
- 2 cloves garlic, pressed
- 2 bell peppers, chopped
- 2 ½ pounds tiger prawns, deveined
- ¼ teaspoon ground black pepper
- 1 teaspoon paprika
- 1 teaspoon red chili flakes
- ½ teaspoon mustard seeds
- ½ teaspoon fennel seeds
- Sea salt, to taste
- ½ cup Marsala wine

1. Heat the olive oil and ghee in a frying pan over a medium-high flame. Now, sweat the scallions, garlic, and peppers until they are crisp-tender about 2 minutes.
2. Add in the tiger prawns and cook for 1 ½ minutes on each side until they are opaque.
3. Stir in the remaining ingredients and continue to cook for 5 minutes more over low heat. Taste and adjust seasonings. Bon appétit!

Per Serving

Calories: **219** | Fat: **6.5g** | Carbs: **2.7g** | Protein: **39g** | Fiber: **0.6g**

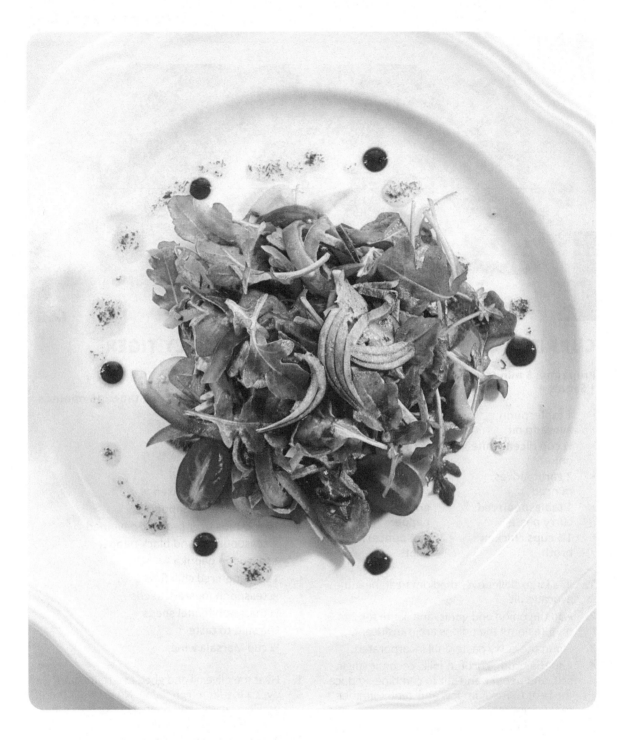

CHAPTER 8: VEGETABLES AND SIDE DISHES

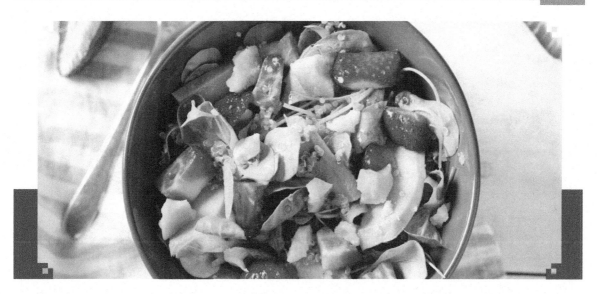

SUNDAY CAULIFLOWER AND HAM BAKE

Prep time: 5 minutes | Cook time: 10 minutes | Serves 6

- 1 ½ pounds cauliflower, broken into small florets
- ½ cup Greek-Style yogurt
- 4 eggs, beaten
- 6 ounces ham, diced
- 1 cup Swiss cheese, preferably freshly grated

1. Place the cauliflower into a deep saucepan; cover with water and bring to a boil over high heat; immediately reduce the heat to medium-low.
2. Let it simmer, covered, approximately 6 minutes. Drain and mash with a potato masher.
3. Add in the yogurt, eggs and ham; stir until everything is well combined and incorporated.
4. Scrape the mixture into a lightly greased casserole dish. Top with the grated Swiss cheese and transfer to a preheated at 390 degrees F oven.
5. Bake for 15 to 20 minutes or until cheese bubbles and browns. Bon appétit!

Per Serving

Calories: 236 | Fat: 13.8g | Carbs: 7.2g | Protein: 20.3g | Fiber: 2.3g

BERRY AVOCADO SALAD

Prep time: 10 minutes | Cook time: 0 minutes | Serves 4

Dressing
- 2 tablespoons extra-virgin olive oil or refined avocado oil
- 1½ teaspoons fresh lime juice
- 1½ teaspoons chili powder
- 1 small clove garlic, minced
- 2 drops liquid stevia
- Finely ground gray sea salt, to taste

Salad
- 2 large Hass avocados, skinned, pitted, and cubed 12 strawberries, cut into quarters or eighths (depending on size)
- ½ packed cup fresh parsley, chopped
- 1 packed tablespoon fresh cilantro leaves, chopped
- 1 tablespoon finely diced white onion

1. Place the ingredients for the dressing in a large bowl and whisk to combine. Add the salad ingredients and toss gently to coat.
2. Divide the salad among 4 bowls and serve immediately.

Per Serving

Calories: 259 | Fat: 21.5g | Carbs: 12.8g | Fiber: 9.9g | Protein: 3.5g

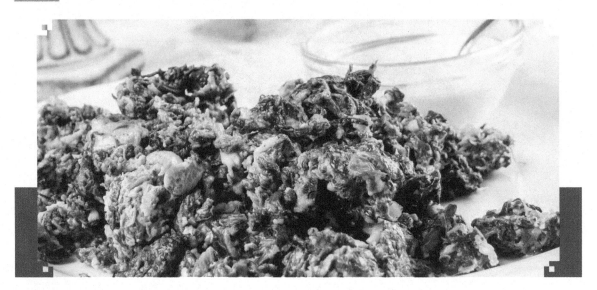

COCONUT CREAMED SPINACH

Prep time: 10 minutes | Cook time: 20 minutes | Serves 4

- 1 tablespoon grass-fed butter
- ¼ onion, thinly sliced
- 4 cups coarsely chopped spinach, thoroughly washed
- ½ cup vegetable broth
- ¼ cup coconut cream
- ⅛ teaspoon ground nutmeg
- Pinch sea salt
- Pinch freshly ground black pepper

1. Cook the onion. In a large skillet over medium heat, melt the butter. Add the onion and sauté until it's softened, about 2 minutes.
2. Cook the spinach. Stir in the spinach, vegetable broth, coconut cream, nutmeg, salt, and pepper and cook, giving it a stir from time to time, until the spinach is tender and the sauce thickens, about 15 minutes.
3. Serve. Put the creamed spinach in a bowl and serve.

Per Serving

Calories: 85 | Fat: 8g | Carbs: 3g | Fiber: 1g | Protein: 1g

CREAMY ROASTED ASPARAGUS SALAD

Prep time: 5 minutes | Cook time: 20 minutes | Serves 5

- 14 ounces asparagus spears, trimmed
- 2 tablespoons olive oil
- ½ teaspoon oregano
- ½ teaspoon rosemary
- Sea salt and freshly ground black pepper, to taste
- 5 tablespoons mayonnaise
- 3 tablespoons sour cream
- 1 tablespoon wine vinegar
- 1 teaspoon fresh garlic, minced
- 1 cup cherry tomatoes, halved

1. In a lightly greased roasting pan, toss the asparagus with the olive oil, oregano, rosemary, salt, and black pepper.
2. Roast in the preheated oven at 425 degrees F for 13 to 15 minutes until just tender.
3. Meanwhile, in a mixing bowl, thoroughly combine the mayonnaise, sour cream, vinegar, and garlic; dress the salad and top with the cherry tomato halves.
4. Serve at room temperature. Bon appétit!

Per Serving

Calories: 179 | Fat: 17.5g | Carbs: 4.7g | Protein: 2.5g | Fiber: 2g

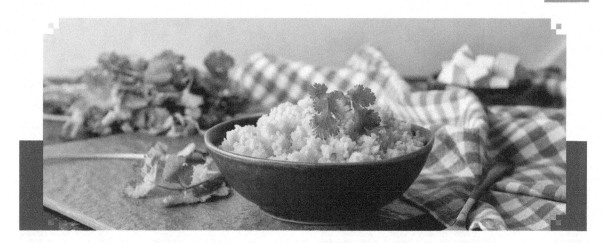

VEGETARIAN PAD THAI

Prep time: **10 minutes** | Cook time: **15 minutes** | Serves **6**

- 2 cups spiral-cut daikon noodles
- 4 cups chopped napa cabbage
- 1 cup chopped red cabbage
- ¼ cup chopped fresh cilantro
- ¼ cup slivered almonds

For the Dressing:

- ½ cup filtered water
- ¼ cup natural almond butter (no sugar added)
- 2 tablespoons peeled and minced fresh ginger
- 1 tablespoon fish sauce (no sugar added) or coconut aminos for strict vegetarian or vegan
- 1 tablespoon granulated erythritol
- 1 tablespoon lime juice
- 1 tablespoon toasted sesame oil
- 1 tablespoon wheat-free soy sauce
- 1 teaspoon minced garlic
- ½ teaspoon kosher salt
- ¼ teaspoon cayenne pepper

1. Combine the daikon noodles, cabbage, cilantro, and almonds in a large bowl.
2. Place the dressing ingredients in a small blender and blend until smooth. Pour the dressing over the vegetables and toss well to coat. Serve immediately.
3. Store any leftovers in an airtight container in the refrigerator for up to 5 days.

Per Serving

Calories: **145** | Fat: **10g** | Protein: **5g** | Carbs: **7g** | Fiber: **3g**

CAULIFLOWER RICE

Prep time: **15 minutes** | Cook time: **15 minutes** | Serves **4**

- ⅓ cup lard
- 4 cups riced cauliflower florets
- 1 cup chicken bone broth
- ½ teaspoon finely ground gray sea salt

1. Place the lard in a large frying pan over medium heat. When melted, add the remaining ingredients. Cover and cook for 8 to 10 minutes, until the rice has softened.
2. Remove the lid and cook for another 5 minutes, or until the liquid has evaporated.
3. Divide the rice among 4 small bowls and serve.

Per Serving

Calories: **200** | Fat: **17.2g** | Carbs: **6.6g** | Fiber: **3.1g** | Protein: **4.6g**

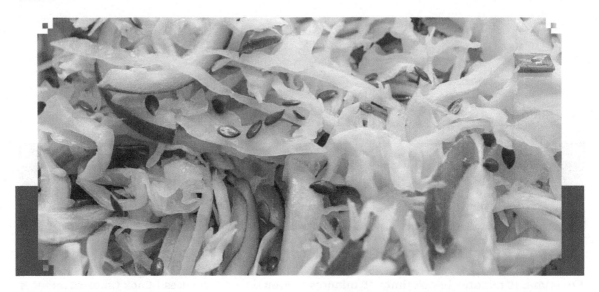

BRUSSELS SPROUT SLAW

Prep time: **15 minutes** | Cook time: **15 minutes** | Serves **4**

- 1 pound Brussels sprouts, stem ends removed and sliced thin
- ½ red onion, sliced thin
- 1 apple, cored and sliced thin
- 1 teaspoon Dijon mustard
- 1 teaspoon salt
- 1 tablespoon raw honey or maple syrup
- 2 teaspoons apple cider vinegar
- 1 cup plain coconut milk yogurt
- ½ cup chopped toasted hazelnuts
- ½ cup pomegranate seeds

1. In a medium bowl, combine the Brussels sprouts, onion, and apple.
2. In a small bowl, whisk together the Dijon mustard, salt, honey, cider vinegar, and yogurt.
3. Add the dressing to the Brussels sprouts and toss until evenly coated.
4. Garnish the salad with the hazelnuts and pomegranate seeds.

Per Serving

Calories: **189** | Fat: **8g** | Carbs: **29g** | Fiber: **9g** | Protein: **6g**

VEGETABLE VODKA SAUCE BAKE

Prep time: **10 minutes** | Cook time: **30 minutes** | Serves **4**

- 3 tablespoons melted grass-fed butter, divided
- 4 cups mushrooms, halved
- 4 cups cooked cauliflower florets
- 1½ cups purchased vodka sauce (see Tip)
- ¾ cup heavy (whipping) cream
- ½ cup grated Asiago cheese
- Sea salt, for seasoning
- Freshly ground black pepper, for seasoning
- 1 cup shredded provolone cheese
- 2 tablespoons chopped fresh oregano

1. Preheat the oven. Set the oven temperature to 350°F and use 1 tablespoon of the melted butter to grease a 9-by-13-inch baking dish.
2. Mix the vegetables. In a large bowl, combine the mushrooms, cauliflower, vodka sauce, cream, Asiago, and the remaining 2 tablespoons of butter. Season the vegetables with salt and pepper.
3. Bake. Transfer the vegetable mixture to the baking dish and top it with the provolone cheese. Bake for 30 to 35 minutes until it's bubbly and heated through.
4. Serve. Divide the mixture between four plates and top with the oregano.

Per Serving

Calories: **537** | Fat: **45g** | Carbs: **14g** | Fiber: **6g** | Protein: **19g**

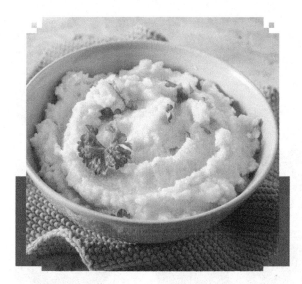 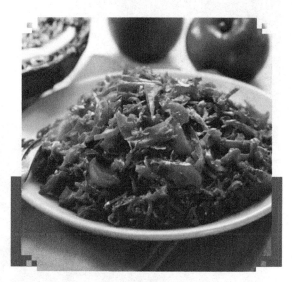

CREAMY CAULIFLOWER MASH

Prep time: **15 minutes** | Cook time: **30 minutes** | Serves **4**

- 1 medium head cauliflower, cut into 1-inch pieces
- 5 cloves garlic
- Needles from 2 sprigs fresh rosemary
- 2 tablespoons bacon fat, melted
- 1 teaspoon fine Himalayan salt
- 1 teaspoon ground black pepper
- ¼ cup coconut cream
- 2 large egg yolks

1. Preheat the oven to 400°F.
2. On a sheet pan, toss the cauliflower pieces with the garlic, rosemary, and bacon fat. Spread them evenly over the pan and roast for 30 minutes, until the cauliflower is toasted and the garlic is golden brown.
3. Transfer the cauliflower, garlic, and rosemary to a food processor. Add the salt and pepper and pulse until the mixture is broken down. Add the coconut cream and egg yolks, then blend until smooth. You might need to stop and scrape down the sides once or twice. The mash will be thick and rich.
4. Serve hot. Store leftovers in the fridge in an airtight container for up to 5 days.

Per Serving

Calories: **171** | Fat: **13g** | Carbs: **10g** | Fiber: **4g** | Protein: **5g**

CREAMY BRAISED KALE

Prep time: **5 minutes** | Cook time: **15 minutes** | Serves **5**

- 1 tablespoons olive oil
- 1 shallot, chopped
- 6 cups kale, torn into pieces
- ½ teaspoon fresh garlic, minced
- 2 tablespoons dry white wine
- ¼ teaspoon red pepper flakes, crushed
- Sea salt and ground black pepper, to taste
- ½ cup double cream

1. Heat the olive oil in a large, heavy-bottomed sauté pan over moderate heat. Now, sauté the shallot until it is tender or about 4 minutes.
2. Stir in the kale and continue to cook for 2 minutes more. Remove any excess liquid and stir in the garlic; continue to cook for a minute or so.
3. Add a splash of wine to deglaze the pan. Then, add the red pepper, salt, black pepper, and double cream to the pan.
4. Turn the heat to simmer. Continue to simmer, covered, for a further 4 minutes. Serve warm and enjoy!

Per Serving

Calories: **130** | Fat: **10.5g** | Carbs: **6.1g** | Protein: **3.7g** | Fiber: **3g**

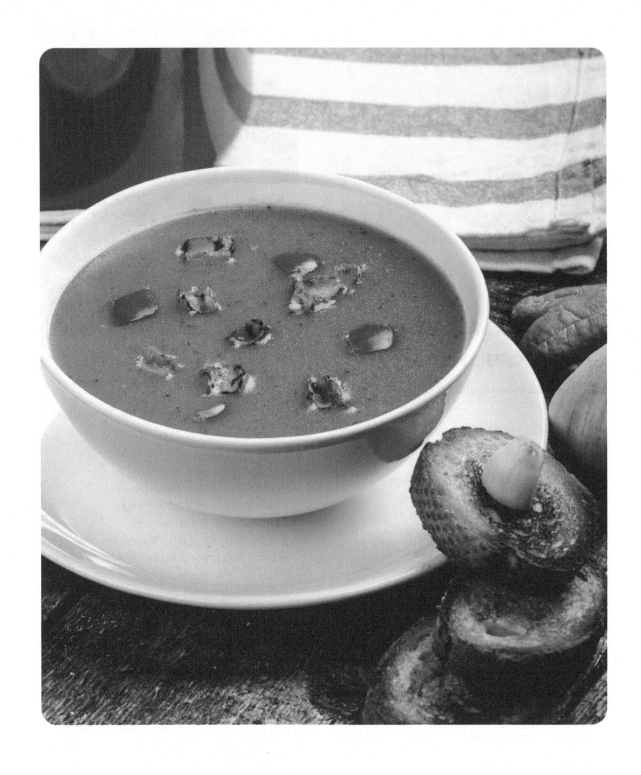

CHAPTER 9: SOUPS AND STEW

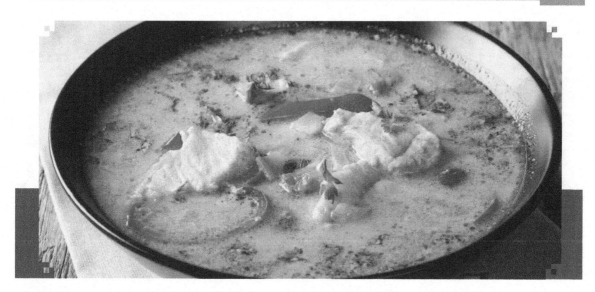

OLD-FASHIONED CHICKEN SOUP

Prep time: **5 minutes** | Cook time: **55 minutes** |Serves **6**

- 1 rotisserie chicken, shredded
- 6 cups water
- 2 tablespoons butter
- 2 celery stalks, chopped
- ½ onion, chopped
- 1 bay leaf
- Sea salt and ground black pepper, to taste
- 1 tablespoon fresh cilantro, chopped
- 2 cups green cabbage, sliced into strips

1. Cook the bones and carcass from a leftover chicken with water over medium-high heat for 15 minutes. Then, reduce to a simmer and cook an additional 15 minutes. Reserve the chicken along with the broth.
2. Let it cool enough to handle, shred the meat into bite-size pieces.
3. Melt the butter in a large stockpot over medium heat. Sauté the celery and onion until tender and fragrant.
4. Add bay leaf, salt, pepper, and broth, and let it simmer for 10 minutes.
5. Add the reserved chicken, cilantro, and cabbage. Simmer for an additional 10 to 11 minutes, until the cabbage is tender. Bon appétit!

Per Serving

Calories: **265** | Fat: **23.8g** | Carbs: **4.3g** | Fiber: **1.7g** | Protein: **9.3g**

COCONUT FISH STEW

Prep time: **15 minutes** | Cook time: **10 minutes** | Serves **4**

- 2 tablespoons coconut oil
- 1 white onion, sliced thin
- 2 garlic cloves, sliced thin
- 2 zucchini, sliced thin
- 1 ½ pounds firm white fish fillet, cut into 1-inch cubes
- 1 (4-inch) piece lemongrass (white part only), bruised with the back of a knife
- 1 (13.5-ounce) can coconut milk
- 1 teaspoon salt
- ¼ teaspoon freshly ground white pepper
- ½ cup slivered scallions
- ¼ cup chopped cilantro
- 3 tablespoons freshly squeezed lemon juice

1. In a large pot over medium heat, melt the coconut oil.
2. Add the onion, garlic, and zucchini. Sauté for 5 minutes.
3. Add the fish, lemongrass, coconut milk, salt, and white pepper to the pot. If the liquid doesn't cover the fish, add enough water to do so. Bring to a boil, then reduce the heat to simmer, and cook for 5 minutes.
4. Garnish the soup with the scallions, cilantro, and lemon juice.

Per Serving

Calories: **608** | Fat: **43g** |Carbs: **13g** | Fiber: **4g** | Protein: **46g**

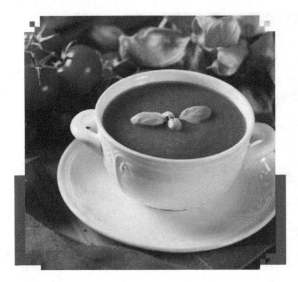

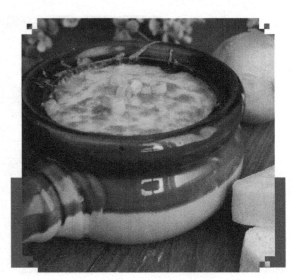

TOMATO SOUP

Prep time: **10 minutes** | Cook time: **15 minutes** | Serves **4**

- 2 tablespoons extra-virgin olive oil
- 1 onion, finely chopped
- 2 garlic cloves, minced
- 2 (28-ounce) cans crushed tomatoes, undrained
- 4 cups no-salt-added vegetable broth
- ½ teaspoon sea salt
- ⅛ teaspoon freshly ground black pepper

1. In a large pot over medium-high heat, heat the olive oil until it shimmers.
2. Add the onion. Cook for about 7 minutes, stirring occasionally, until browned.
3. Add the garlic. Cook for 30 seconds, stirring constantly.
4. Stir in the tomatoes, vegetable broth, salt, and pepper. Simmer for 5 minutes.
5. Carefully transfer the soup to a blender or use an immersion blender. Process until smooth.

Per Serving

Calories: **233** | Fat: **7g** | Carbs: **35g** | Fiber: **13g** | Protein: **10g**

CLASSIC FRENCH ONION SOUP

Prep time: **15 minutes** | Cook time: **2 hours, 30 minutes** | Serves **4**

- 2 tablespoons olive oil
- 3 pounds sweet onions, halved and cut into ⅛-inch-thick slices (a mandoline or food processor slicing disc helps here)
- 2 teaspoons bottled minced garlic
- ½ cup dry sherry
- 8 cups Beef Bone Broth
- 1 tablespoon chopped fresh thyme
- Sea salt
- Freshly ground black pepper

1. Place a large stockpot over low heat and add the olive oil.
2. Add the onions and garlic. Cover the pot and cook for 30 minutes, letting the juices purge from the onions. Stir occasionally.
3. Remove the lid. Continue to sauté the onions and garlic, stirring occasionally, for about 1 hour, 30 minutes, or until they are a deep caramel color.
4. Add the sherry and deglaze the pan, scraping up any browned bits from the bottom.
5. Increase the heat to medium. Stir in the beef broth and thyme. Bring the soup to a boil. Reduce the heat to low and simmer for about 30 minutes, or until the onions are tender.
6. Season with sea salt and pepper.

Per Serving

Calories: **234** | Fat: **9g** | Carbs: **33g** | Fiber: **8g** | Protein: **9g**

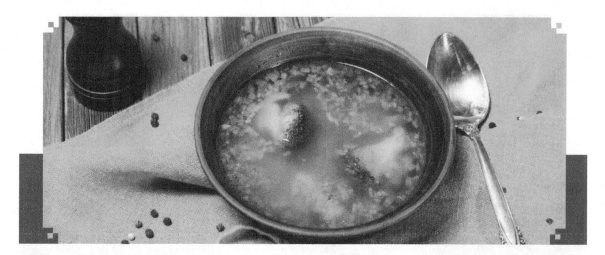

HEARTY PORK STEW

Prep time: **5 minutes** | Cook time: **1 hour** |Serves **5**

- 2 tablespoons olive oil
- 2 pounds pork stew meat
- 1 yellow onion, chopped
- 2 garlic cloves, minced
- ¼ cup dry sherry wine
- 4 cups chicken bone broth
- 1 cup tomatoes, pureed
- 1 bay laurel
- Sea salt and ground black pepper, to taste
- 2 tablespoons fresh cilantro, chopped

1. Heat the olive oil in a soup pot over a moderate flame. Sear the pork for about 5 minutes, stirring continuously to ensure even cooking; reserve.
2. Cook the yellow onion in the pan drippings until just tender and translucent. Stir in the garlic and continue to sauté for a further 30 seconds.
3. Pour in a splash of dry sherry to deglaze the pan.
4. Pour in the chicken bone broth and bring to a boil. Stir in the tomatoes and bay laurel. Season with salt and pepper to taste. Turn the heat to medium-low and continue to cook 10 minutes longer.
5. Add the reserved pork back to the pot, partially cover, and continue to simmer for 45
6. minutes longer. Garnish with cilantro and serve hot. Bon appétit!

Per Serving

Calories:332 | Fat:14.7g | Carbs: 3.9g | Protein: 41g | Fiber:0.8g

BROCCOLI AND LENTIL STEW

Prep time: **15 minutes** | Cook time: **30 minutes** | Serves **4**

- 1 tablespoon extra-virgin olive oil, plus additional for drizzling
- 1 small onion, finely chopped
- 1 small carrot, chopped
- 2 cloves garlic, minced
- 2 cups vegetable broth
- 1 cup dried green or brown lentils
- 1 teaspoon dried oregano
- 6 cups broccoli florets
- 1 teaspoon salt
- ¼ teaspoon freshly ground black pepper
- ½ cup sliced pitted green olives
- ¼ cup chopped fresh Italian parsley

1. In a large pot over high heat, heat the olive oil.
2. Add the onion, carrot, and garlic. Sauté for 5 minutes.
3. Add the vegetable broth, lentils, and oregano and bring to a boil. Reduce the heat to simmer. Cook the soup for 15 to 20 minutes, or until the lentils are tender.
4. Add the broccoli, cover the pot, and simmer for 5 minutes more.
5. Remove the pot from the heat and stir in the olives and parsley. If the soup is too thick, stir in some water.
6. Ladle the soup into bowls, drizzle with a little olive oil, and serve.

Per Serving

Calories: **182** | Fat: **6g** |Carbs: **24g** | Fiber: **9g** | Protein: **11g**

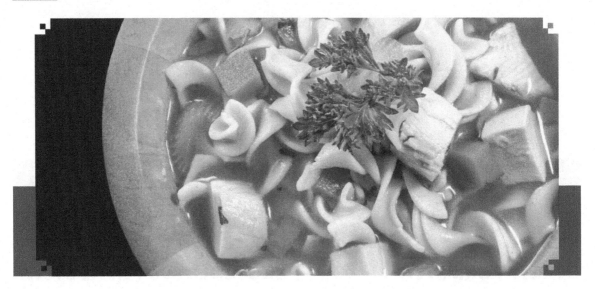

CHILI-INFUSED LAMB SOUP

Prep time: 5 minutes | Cook time: 25 minutes | Serves 6

- 1 tablespoon coconut oil
- ¾ pound ground lamb
- 2 cups shredded cabbage
- ½ onion, chopped
- 2 teaspoons minced garlic
- 4 cups chicken broth
- 2 cups coconut milk
- 1½ tablespoons red chili paste or as much as you want
- Zest and juice of 1 lime
- 1 cup shredded kale

1. Cook the lamb. In a medium stockpot over medium-high heat, warm the coconut oil. Add the lamb and cook it, stirring it often, until it has browned, about 6 minutes.
2. Cook the vegetables. Add the cabbage, onion, and garlic and sauté until they've softened, about 5 minutes.
3. Simmer the soup. Stir in the chicken broth, coconut milk, red chili paste, lime zest, and lime juice. Bring it to a boil, then reduce the heat to low and simmer until the cabbage is tender, about 10 minutes.
4. Add the kale. Stir in the kale and simmer the soup for 3 more minutes.
5. Serve. Spoon the soup into six bowls and serve.

Per Serving

Calories: 380 | Fat: 32g | Carbs: 7g | Fiber: 1g | Protein: 17g

CHICKEN NOODLE SOUP

Prep time: 10 minutes | Cook time: 35 minutes | Serves 4

- ⅓ cup coconut oil or duck fat
- 1 pound boneless, skinless chicken thighs, sliced
- 1 cup diced celery
- 1 cup chopped green onions, green parts only
- ½ cup diced carrots
- 6 cups chicken bone broth
- 2 teaspoons finely ground gray sea salt
- ½ teaspoon dried basil
- ½ teaspoon dried oregano leaves
- ⅛ teaspoon ground black pepper
- 2 cups noodles

1. Heat the oil in a large saucepan over medium-high heat, then add the sliced chicken. Brown the chicken on both sides, about 10 minutes total.
2. Add the celery, onions, and carrots to the pan and continue to cook for 5 minutes.
3. Add the broth, salt, basil, oregano, and pepper. Cover and bring to a boil. Once boiling, reduce the heat to medium-low and cook for 20 minutes. In the last 2 minutes of cooking, add the noodles.
4. Remove from the heat and divide the soup among 4 medium-sized serving bowls.

Per Serving

Calories: 371 | Fat: 22.2g | Carbs: 6.5g | Fiber: 2.3g | Protein: 36.4g

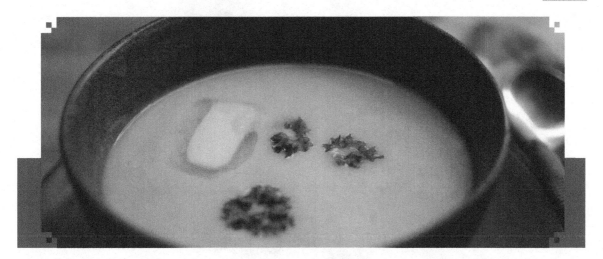

CHICKEN FENNEL SOUP

Prep time: **20 minutes** | Cook time: **45 minutes** | Serves 4

- 1 tablespoon olive oil
- 1 sweet onion, chopped, or about 1 cup precut packaged onion
- 2 teaspoons bottled minced garlic
- 3 cups shredded fennel
- 3 cups shredded green cabbage, or packaged shredded cabbage (see Tip)
- 2 carrots, chopped, or about 1 cup precut packaged carrots
- 8 cups Herbed Chicken Bone Broth
- 2 teaspoons chopped fresh thyme
- 2 cups chopped cooked chicken breast
- Pinch sea salt

1. Place a large stockpot over medium-high heat and add the olive oil.
2. Add the onion and garlic. Sauté for about 3 minutes, or until the onion is translucent.
3. Stir in the fennel, cabbage, and carrots. Sauté for about 5 minutes, or until the vegetables have softened.
4. Stir in the chicken broth and thyme. Bring the soup to a boil. Reduce the heat to low and simmer for about 30 minutes, or until the vegetables are tender.
5. Add the chicken and sea salt. Simmer for about 5 minutes, or until the chicken is heated through.

Per Serving

Calories: **255** | Fat: **10g** | Carbs: **16g** | Fiber: **5g** | Protein: **25g**

CHEESY CAULIFLOWER SOUP

Prep time: **5 minutes** | Cook time: **20 minutes** | Serves 4

- ½ onion, chopped
- 2 cups riced/shredded cauliflower (I buy it pre-riced at Trader Joe's)
- 1 cup chicken broth
- 2 ounces cream cheese
- 1 cup heavy (whipping) cream
- Pink Himalayan salt
- Freshly ground pepper
- ½ cup shredded Cheddar cheese (I use sharp Cheddar)

1. In a medium saucepan over medium heat, melt the butter. Add the onion and cook, stirring occasionally, until softened, about 5 minutes.
2. Add the cauliflower and chicken broth, and allow the mixture to come to a boil, stirring occasionally.
3. Lower the heat to medium-low and simmer until the cauliflower is soft enough to mash, about 10 minutes.
4. Add the cream cheese, and mash the mixture.
5. Add the cream and purée the mixture with an immersion blender (or you can pour the soup into the blender, blend it, and then pour it back into the pan and reheat it a bit).
6. Season the soup with pink Himalayan salt and pepper.
7. Pour the soup into four bowls, top each with the shredded Cheddar cheese, and serve.

Per Serving

Calories: **372** | Fat: **35g** | Carbs: **9g** | Fiber: **3g** | Protein: **9g**

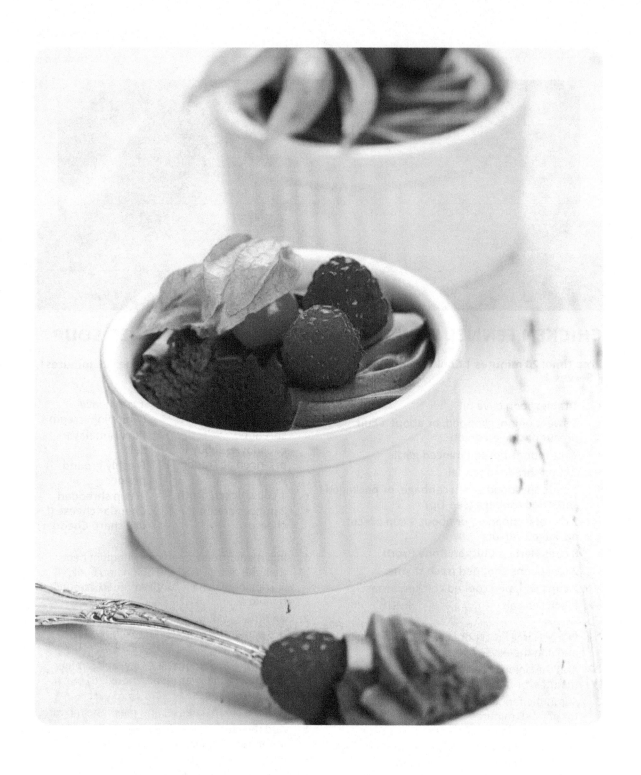

CHAPTER 10:
DESSERTS

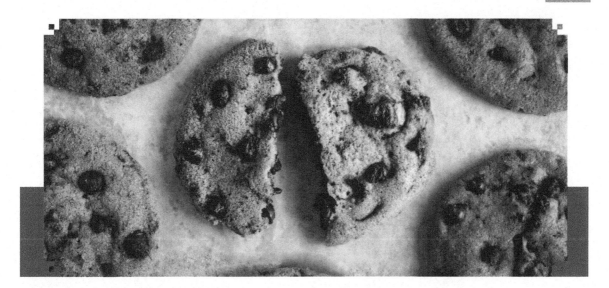

CHEWY DOUBLE CHOCOLATE CHIP COOKIES

Prep time: 15 minutes | Cook time: 10 minutes | Serves 4

- ¾ cup creamy almond butter
- ½ cup coconut sugar
- ¼ cup cocoa powder
- 2 teaspoons vanilla extract
- 1 egg
- 1 egg yolk
- 1 teaspoon baking soda
- ¼ teaspoon salt
- ½ cup semi-sweet chocolate chips
- Dash sea salt (optional)

1. Preheat the oven to 350°F.
2. Line 2 baking sheets with parchment paper.
3. In a medium bowl, cream together the almond butter, coconut sugar, cocoa powder, and vanilla.
4. In a small bowl, whisk the egg and egg yolk. Add the eggs to the almond butter mixture, and stir to combine.
5. Stir in the baking soda, salt, and chocolate chips until well mixed. Divide the dough into 12 pieces. Roll the dough into balls and put 6 on each prepared pan.
6. Bake for 9 to 10 minutes. Let the cookies rest on the pans for 5 minutes, where they'll continue to cook. Sprinkle each with a dash of sea salt (if using). Remove to a cooling rack.

Per Serving

Calories: 226 | Fat: 15g | Carbs: 20g | Fiber: 3g; | Protein: 6g

BLUEBERRY-PEACH COBBLER

Prep time: 15 minutes | Cook time: 2 hours | Serves 4 to 6

- 5 tablespoons coconut oil, divided
- 3 large peaches, peeled and sliced
- 2 cups frozen blueberries
- 1 cup almond flour
- 1 cup rolled oats
- 1 tablespoon maple syrup
- 1 tablespoon coconut sugar
- 1 teaspoon ground cinnamon
- ½ teaspoon vanilla extract
- Pinch ground nutmeg

1. Coat the bottom of your slow cooker with 1 tablespoon of coconut oil.
2. Arrange the peaches and blueberries along the bottom of the slow cooker.
3. In a small bowl, stir together the almond flour, oats, remaining 4 tablespoons of coconut oil, maple syrup, coconut sugar, cinnamon, vanilla, and nutmeg until a coarse mixture forms. Gently crumble the topping over the fruit in the slow cooker.
4. Cover the cooker and set to high. Cook for 2 hours and serve.

Per Serving

Calories: 516 | Fat: 34g |Carbs: 49g |Fiber: 10g | Protein: 10g

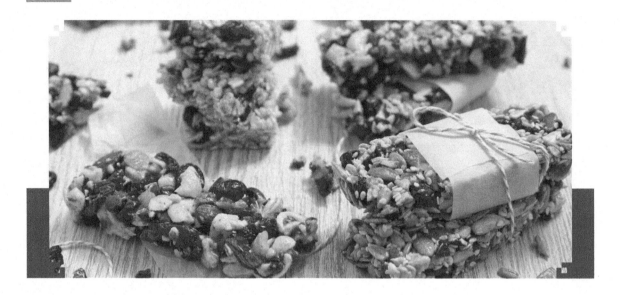

GLUTEN-FREE OAT AND FRUIT BARS

Prep time: 15 minutes | Cook time: 40-45 minutes | Makes 16 bars

- Cooking spray
- ½ cup maple syrup
- ½ cup almond or sunflower butter
- 2 medium ripe bananas, mashed
- ⅓ cup dried cranberries
- 1½ cups old-fashioned rolled oats
- ½ cup shredded coconut
- ¼ cup oat flour
- ¼ cup ground flaxseed
- 1 teaspoon vanilla extract
- ½ teaspoon ground cinnamon
- ¼ teaspoon ground cloves

1. Preheat the oven to 400°F.
2. Line an 8-by-8-inch square pan with parchment paper or aluminum foil, and coat the lined pan with cooking spray.
3. In a medium bowl, combine the maple syrup, almond butter, and bananas. Mix until well blended.
4. Add the cranberries, oats, coconut, oat flour, flaxseed, vanilla, cinnamon, and cloves. Mix well.
5. Spoon the mixture into the prepared pan; the mixture will be thick and sticky. Use an oiled spatula to spread the mixture evenly.
6. Place the pan in the preheated oven and bake for 40 to 45 minutes, or until the top is dry and a toothpick inserted in the middle comes out clean. Cool completely before cutting into bars.

Per Serving

Calories: 144 | Fat: 7g |Carbs: 19g | Fiber: 2g | Protein: 3g

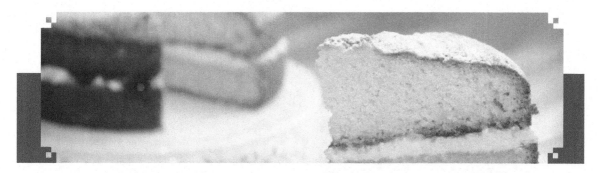

TENDER COCONUT CAKE

Prep time: **15 minutes** | Cook time: **45 minutes** | Serves **8**

- ½ cup coconut oil, melted, plus more for greasing the baking dish
- 2 cups egg whites (about 12), at room temperature
- Pinch sea salt
- 1 cup unsweetened almond milk
- 6 tablespoons raw honey
- 2 teaspoons pure vanilla extract
- 1 cup coconut flour
- ½ cup shredded unsweetened coconut
- 2 teaspoons baking powder

1. Preheat the oven to 350°F.
2. Lightly grease a 9-by-13-inch baking dish with coconut oil and set it aside.
3. In a large bowl, beat the egg whites and sea salt with an electric mixer until soft peaks form. Set them aside.
4. In another large bowl, whisk the almond milk, honey, remaining ½ cup of coconut oil, and the vanilla.
5. Whisk in the coconut flour, coconut, and baking powder until well combined.
6. Fold the beaten egg whites into the batter, keeping as much volume as possible, until just blended. Spoon the batter into the prepared dish and smooth the top.
7. Bake the cake for about 45 minutes, or until cooked through and lightly browned.
8. Cool the cake completely on a wire rack.
9. Serve with fresh fruit, if desired.

Per Serving

Calories: **237** | Fat: **17g** | Carbs: **16g** | Fiber: **1g** | Protein: **7g**

POPPY SEED POUND CAKE

Prep time: **10 minutes** | Cook time: **40 minutes** | Serves **12**

- 4 tablespoons (½ stick) unsalted butter, at room temperature, plus more for greasing
- 1¼ cups finely milled almond flour, sifted
- 1 teaspoon baking powder
- ¼ teaspoon salt
- ¾ cup granulated erythritol–monk fruit blend; less sweet: ½ cup
- 3½ ounces full-fat cream cheese, at room temperature
- 1 teaspoon lemon extract
- 4 large eggs, at room temperature
- 1½ tablespoons poppy seeds

1. Preheat the oven to 350°F. Grease the loaf pan with butter, line with parchment paper, and set aside.
2. In the medium bowl, combine the almond flour, baking powder, and salt. Set aside.
3. In the large bowl, using an electric mixer on medium high, cream the butter and erythritol–monk fruit blend for 1 to 2 minutes, until light and fluffy.
4. Add the cream cheese and lemon extract and mix well. Add the eggs, one at a time, making sure to mix well after each addition. Add the dry ingredients to the wet ingredients and mix well. Stir in the poppy seeds and mix well.
5. Pour the batter into the prepared loaf pan. Bake for 30 to 40 minutes, until golden brown and a toothpick inserted into the center comes out clean. Let cool for 10 to 15 minutes, then cut into 12 slices and serve.
6. Store leftovers in an airtight container in the refrigerator for up to 5 days or freeze for up to 3 weeks.

Per Serving

Calories: **149** | Fat: **14g** | Carbs: **3g** | Fiber: **2g** | Protein: **5g**

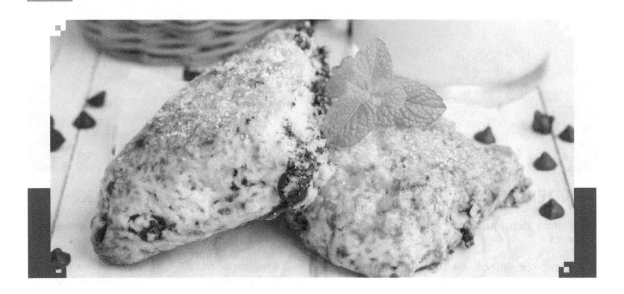

CHOCOLATE CHIP SCONES

Prep time:10 minutes | Cook time: 30 minutes | Serves 10

- 4 tablespoons (½ stick) unsalted butter, melted, plus more for greasing
- ½ cup granulated erythritol–monk fruit blend
- 3 large eggs
- ½ cup full-fat sour cream
- 1½ cups finely milled almond flour, sifted
- ½ cup coconut flour
- 1½ teaspoons baking powder
- ¼ teaspoon sea salt
- 4 ounces sugar-free chocolate chips
- 2 tablespoons confectioners' erythritol– monk fruit blend, for dusting (optional)

1. Preheat the oven to 375°F. Grease the cast-iron skillet with butter and set aside.
2. In the large bowl, using an electric mixer on medium high, mix the granulated erythritol–monk fruit blend, melted butter, and eggs until well combined, stopping and scraping the bowl once or twice, as needed. Add the sour cream and mix well. Add the almond flour, coconut flour, baking powder, and salt, then stir until fully combined. Fold the sugar-free chocolate chips into the batter.
3. Spread the batter evenly into the cast-iron skillet. Bake for 25 to 30 minutes, or until a toothpick inserted into the center comes out clean. Allow the scones to cool completely. Dust with confectioners' erythritol–monk fruit blend (if using) and cut into 10 wedges before serving.
4. Store leftovers in an airtight container in the refrigerator for up to 5 days or freeze for up to 3 weeks.

Per Serving

Calories: 268 | Fat: 24g |Carbs: 8g |Fiber: 4g | Protein: 7g

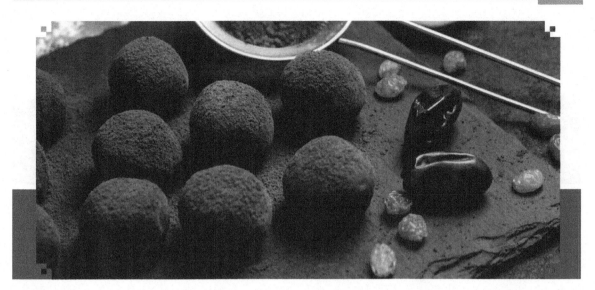

LEMON COCONUT TRUFFLES

Prep time: 30 minutes | Cook time: 5 minutes | Serves 4

- 3 cups shredded unsweetened coconut, divided
- ½ cup pecans
- 2 tablespoons coconut oil
- Zest and juice of 1 lemon
- ½ cup monk fruit sweetener, granulated form
- Pinch sea salt

1. Make the truffle base. Put 2 cups of the coconut and the pecans in a food processor and pulse until the mixture looks like a paste, about 5 minutes.
2. Add the remaining ingredients. Add the coconut oil, lemon zest, lemon juice, sweetener, and salt to the processor and pulse until the mixture forms a big ball, about 2 minutes.
3. Form the truffles. Scoop the mixture out with a tablespoon and roll it into 16 balls. Roll the truffles in the remaining 1 cup of coconut.
4. Store. Store the truffles in a sealed container in the refrigerator for up to one week or in the freezer for up to one month.

Per Serving

Calories: 160 | Fat: 16g | Carbs: 5g | Fiber: 3g | Protein: 2g

HONEYED APPLE CINNAMON COMPOTE

Prep time: 15 minutes | Cook time: 10 minutes | Serves 4

- 6 apples, peeled, cored, and chopped
- ¼ cup apple juice
- ¼ cup honey
- 1 teaspoon ground cinnamon
- Pinch sea salt

1. In a large pot over medium-high heat, combine the apples, apple juice, honey, cinnamon, and salt.
2. Simmer for about 10 minutes, stirring occasionally, until the apples are still quite chunky but also saucy.

Per Serving

Calories: 247 | Fat: <1g |Carbs: 66g | Fiber: 9g | Protein: 1g

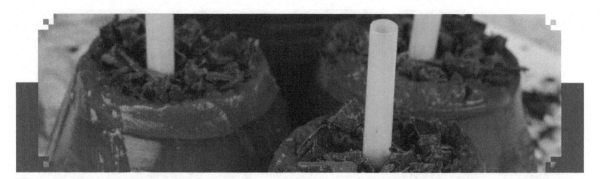

CHOCOLATE-DIPPED PEANUT BUTTER ICE POPS

Prep time: **10 minutes** | **Cook time: 5 minutes** | **Serves 12**

- 8 ounces full-fat cream cheese, at room temperature
- 1 cup all-natural peanut butter (no added sugar or salt)
- ¼ cup confectioners' erythritol–monk fruit blend; less sweet: 2 tablespoons
- 1 teaspoon vanilla extract
- ¼ teaspoon sea salt
- 2 cups heavy (whipping) cream
- 4 ounces sugar-free chocolate chips
- 2 tablespoons coconut oil

1. In the large bowl, using an electric mixer on medium high, beat the cream cheese, peanut butter, confectioners' erythritol–monk fruit blend, vanilla, and salt. Add the heavy cream and combine until well incorporated.
2. Pour the mixture into the popsicle molds and add the popsicle sticks. Freeze for 3 to 4 hours, until frozen solid.
3. In the microwave-safe bowl, melt the chocolate baking chips and coconut oil in the microwave in 30-second intervals. Cool for 5 to 10 minutes.
4. Line the baking sheet with parchment paper. Dip the unmolded pops halfway into the melted chocolate, then place them on the prepared sheet and return them to the freezer for about 20 minutes. Store in the freezer in an airtight (nonglass) container for up to 3 weeks.

Per Serving

Calories: 405 | **Fat: 37g** | **Carbs: 9g** | **Fiber: 3g** | **Protein: 9g**

WARM CINNAMON-TURMERIC ALMOND MILK

Prep time: 15 minutes | **Cook time: 3 to 4 hours** | **Serves 4 to 6**

- 4 cups unsweetened almond milk
- 4 cinnamon sticks
- 2 tablespoons coconut oil
- 1 (4-inch) piece turmeric root, roughly chopped
- 1 (2-inch) piece fresh ginger, roughly chopped
- 1 teaspoon raw honey, plus more to taste

1. In your slow cooker, combine the almond milk, cinnamon sticks, coconut oil, turmeric, and ginger.
2. Cover the cooker and set to low. Cook for 3 to 4 hours.
3. Pour the contents of the cooker through a fine-mesh sieve into a clean container; discard the solids.
4. Starting with just 1 teaspoon, add raw honey to taste.

Per Serving

Calories: 133 | **Fat: 11g** | **Carbs: 10g** | **Fiber: 1g** | **Protein: 1g**

MEASUREMENT CONVERSION CHART

VOLUME EQUIVALENTS(DRY)

US STANDARD	METRIC (APPROXIMATE)
1/8 teaspoon	0.5 mL
1/4 teaspoon	1 mL
1/2 teaspoon	2 mL
3/4 teaspoon	4 mL
1 teaspoon	5 mL
1 tablespoon	15 mL
1/4 cup	59 mL
1/2 cup	118 mL
3/4 cup	177 mL
1 cup	235 mL
2 cups	475 mL
3 cups	700 mL
4 cups	1 L

VOLUME EQUIVALENTS(LIQUID)

US STANDARD	US STANDARD (OUNCES)	METRIC (APPROXIMATE)
2 tablespoons	1 fl.oz.	30 mL
1/4 cup	2 fl.oz.	60 mL
1/2 cup	4 fl.oz.	120 mL
1 cup	8 fl.oz.	240 mL
1 1/2 cup	12 fl.oz.	355 mL
2 cups or 1 pint	16 fl.oz.	475 mL
4 cups or 1 quart	32 fl.oz.	1 L
1 gallon	128 fl.oz.	4 L

TEMPERATURES EQUIVALENTS

FAHRENHEIT(F)	CELSIUS(C) (APPROXIMATE)
225 °F	107 °C
250 °F	120 °C
275 °F	135 °C
300 °F	150 °C
325 °F	160 °C
350 °F	180 °C
375 °F	190 °C
400 °F	205 °C
425 °F	220 °C
450 °F	235 °C
475 °F	245 °C
500 °F	260 °C

WEIGHT EQUIVALENTS

US STANDARD	METRIC (APPROXIMATE)
1 ounce	28 g
2 ounces	57 g
5 ounces	142 g
10 ounces	284 g
15 ounces	425 g
16 ounces (1 pound)	455 g
1.5 pounds	680 g
2 pounds	907 g

The Dirty Dozen and Clean Fifteen

The Environmental Working Group (EWG) is a nonprofit, nonpartisan organization dedicated to protecting human health and the environment Its mission is to empower people to live healthier lives in a healthier environment. This organization publishes an annual list of the twelve kinds of produce, in sequence, that have the highest amount of pesticide residue-the Dirty Dozen-as well as a list of the fifteen kinds ofproduce that have the least amount of pesticide residue-the Clean Fifteen.

THE DIRTY DOZEN	THE CLEAN FIFTEEN
• The 2016 Dirty Dozen includes the following produce. These are considered among the year's most important produce to buy organic:	• The least critical to buy organically are the Clean Fifteen list. The following are on the 2016 list:

THE DIRTY DOZEN		THE CLEAN FIFTEEN	
Strawberries	Spinach	Avocados	Papayas
Apples	Tomatoes	Corn	Kiw
Nectarines	Bell peppers	Pineapples	Eggplant
Peaches	Cherry tomatoes	Cabbage	Honeydew
Celery	Cucumbers	Sweet peas	Grapefruit
Grapes	Kale/collard greens	Onions	Cantaloupe
Cherries	Hot peppers	Asparagus	Cauliflower
		Mangos	

THE DIRTY DOZEN	THE CLEAN FIFTEEN
• *The Dirty Dozen list contains two additional itemskale/collard greens and hot peppers-because they tend to contain trace levels of highly hazardous pesticides.*	• *Some of the sweet corn sold in the United States are made from genetically engineered (GE) seedstock. Buy organic varieties of these crops to avoid GE produce.*

APPENDIX 3: INDEX

Hey there!

Wow, can you believe we've reached the end of this culinary journey together? I'm truly thrilled and filled with joy as I think back on all the recipes we've shared and the flavors we've discovered. This experience, blending a bit of tradition with our own unique twists, has been a journey of love for good food. And knowing you've been out there, giving these dishes a try, has made this adventure incredibly special to me.

Even though we're turning the last page of this book, I hope our conversation about all things delicious doesn't have to end. I cherish your thoughts, your experiments, and yes, even those moments when things didn't go as planned. Every piece of feedback you share is invaluable, helping to enrich this experience for us all.

I'd be so grateful if you could take a moment to share your thoughts with me, be it through a review on Amazon or any other place you feel comfortable expressing yourself online. Whether it's praise, constructive criticism, or even an idea for how we might do things differently in the future, your input is what truly makes this journey meaningful.

This book is a piece of my heart, offered to you with all the love and enthusiasm I have for cooking. But it's your engagement and your words that elevate it to something truly extraordinary.

Thank you from the bottom of my heart for being such an integral part of this culinary adventure. Your openness to trying new things and sharing your experiences has been the greatest gift.

Catch you later,

Marilyn R. Holland

Made in the USA
Monee, IL
08 December 2024